Chasing the Intact M

Chasing the Intact Mind

How the Severely Autistic and Intellectually Disabled Were Excluded from the Debates That Affect Them Most

Amy S. F. Lutz

OXFORD
UNIVERSITY PRESS

OXFORD
UNIVERSITY PRESS

Oxford University Press is a department of the University of Oxford. It furthers the University's objective of excellence in research, scholarship, and education by publishing worldwide. Oxford is a registered trade mark of Oxford University Press in the UK and certain other countries.

Published in the United States of America by Oxford University Press
198 Madison Avenue, New York, NY 10016, United States of America.

Library of Congress Cataloging-in-Publication Data
Names: Lutz, Amy S. F., 1970– author.
Title: Chasing the intact mind : how the severely autistic and intellectually disabled were excluded from the debates that affect them most / by Amy S. F. Lutz.
Description: New York, NY : Oxford University Press, [2024] |
Includes bibliographical references and index. |
Identifiers: LCCN 2023012182 (print) | LCCN 2023012183 (ebook) |
ISBN 9780197683842 (hardback) | ISBN 9780197683866 (epub) | ISBN 9780197683873
Subjects: LCSH: Autistic people—Social conditions. |
Autistic people—Biography. | Developmentally disabled—Social conditions. |
Developmentally disabled—Biography. | Parents of autistic children—
Biography—History and criticism. | Parents of developmentally
disabled children—Biography—History and criticism.
Classification: LCC HV1570.23.L88 2024 (print) | LCC HV1570.23 (ebook) |
DDC 616.85/882—dc23/eng/20230511
LC record available at https://lccn.loc.gov/2023012182
LC ebook record available at https://lccn.loc.gov/2023012183

DOI: 10.1093/oso/9780197683842.001.0001

Printed by Sheridan Books, Inc., United States of America

For all those who fight to make the world a better place for the severely autistic and their families, especially my oldest and closest partners in advocacy: Jill Escher, Alison Singer, Gloria Satriale, Lisa Parles, Judith Ursitti, Lee Wachtel, Denise Lombardi, Denise Resnik, and Alycia Halladay. So grateful for your tireless effort, your fearless tenacity, and your unwavering faith in the possibility of a brighter future.
And for Feda Almaliti, whose memory inspires me every day.

Contents

Acknowledgments

I have been privileged to receive indispensable feedback and encouragement at every stage of this project. Particular thanks to Beth Linker for her extraordinarily generous mentorship throughout my years as a doctoral student in the History and Sociology of Sciences department at Penn. Robby Aronowitz, Jonathan Moreno, Jonathan Sadowsky, Meggie Crnic, Jason Chernesky, Anna Mueser, Katie Beals, and Erika Lutz also provided thoughtful comments on this manuscript, for which I'm very grateful.

Thanks to the Minnesota 14(c) providers who took the time to speak with me about their programs: John Wayne Barker, Lori Schluttenhofer, and Laura Johnson. Special thanks to the families who shared their stories about employment and guardianship: Debbie, Marc, and Lisa K.; Mindy, Jack, and Alex S.; Carl, Gail, and Eddie K.; Jane and Jocelyn K.; Leslie and Nick F.; Rebecca J., Abby P., Kate R., and Tracy C.

Thanks to my agent, Jessica Papin, for believing in this work and finding it the perfect home, and thanks as well as to Sarah Harrington and the Oxford University Press team for giving it a place in the world.

But none of this ever would have happened without the extraordinary support of my husband Andy and kids Jonah, Erika, Hilary, Aaron, and Gretchen. Thank you for selflessly giving me the tremendous amount of time I needed, understanding when I couldn't be in two places at once no matter how much I wanted to, and, most importantly, cheering me on—not just while I was writing this book, but always.

Introduction

In her 2006 memoir *Strange Son*, Portia Iversen coined the phrase "intact mind" to describe the typical cognitive abilities she believed were buried within even the most seemingly impaired autistic individuals, like her son Dov—who, at nine years old, was completely nonverbal and spent much of his time "chewing on blocks and tapping stones." Although he didn't know the alphabet, colors, or numbers; although he "could hardly point or nod his head to show what he meant"; although doctors had diagnosed Dov as "retarded" and told Iversen she "shouldn't wreck [her] marriage and destroy [her] other children's lives for his sake, when doing so was utterly and completely useless"—although all these things were true about her son, Iversen still imagined him "falling down a deep well, believed to be dead. And then years later, a light shone down that dark shaft and I could see him there, *somehow still alive*" (emphasis in original).[1]

Iversen may have been the first to use the term "intact mind," but the sentiment itself was not new. Since Clara Claiborne Park described the successful and titular "siege" she staged to free her daughter Jessy from the grip of autism in 1967, this concept has appeared under different names in many of the most popular parent memoirs. I just as easily could have adopted one of the phrases used by other authors, such as the "real child,"[2] the "normal child,"[3] the "intelligent child trapped inside,"[4] or the visually apt but prohibitively wordy "person locked inside a closet at the top of a collapsed stairway, in a boarded-up house that's hidden by overgrown vines, down a driveway blocked by deadfall on a street bypassed by the highway."[5] A close runner-up to "intact mind," for me, was psychologist Bryna Siegel's articulation of the "homunculus theory" in autism, which "holds that inside each intellectually disabled child with autism there is a normally developed being."[6] Ultimately, I chose "intact mind" because I thought that it best, and most efficiently, captured both the profound hopes of parents and the massive stakes for their children's indeterminate futures.

To clarify, the intact mind is not necessarily one that is indistinguishable from a neurotypical mind—although many of these memoirs do end with children losing their autism diagnoses. Particularly in more recent narratives, parents celebrate the quirky differences that remain even after the intact mind has been recovered. Rupert Isaacson notes, at the conclusion of his 2009 memoir, "Rowan is still autistic—his essence, his many talents, are all tied up with it."[7] And Lori Ashley Taylor proudly quotes her daughter Hannah's observation that she is "'like a Skittle in a Mason jar full of M&Ms.'"[8] These accounts echo claims of autism exceptionality most famously made by autistic adult Temple Grandin, who rhetorically asked, "Who figured out how to make the first stone spear? It wasn't the yakkity yaks [neurotypicals], that's for sure. It was some Asperger sitting in the back of a cave figuring out how to chip rocks into spearheads."[9]

The critical elements of the intact mind are its innateness, integrity, and inaccessibility—at least at first. In other words, there is a profound disjunct between the child's inappropriate, destructive, or even aggressive behaviors and the capable self that has always been hidden deep inside. Barry Neil Kaufman, for example, describes the "vast field of intelligence that we felt existed beneath the surface of [his son Raun's] bizarre patterns";[10] Catherine Maurice sees her daughter Anne-Marie as "'walled-in'" by her autism and is determined to "assaul[t] those ramparts";[11] Robert Hughes writes of "the normal boy hidden just under the silent surface"[12] of his son Walker; Judy Barron recounts, "We caught rare and fleeting glimpses of a helpless child trapped inside the bizarre behavior of Sean's autism, and we were determined to get him out. . . . Sean and I have written the story of his release from the terrifying imprisonment of his own mind."[13]

As the mother of an autistic son[14] who was born in 1999 and diagnosed at the age of two, I too was terrified. Terrified—but inspired, and determined never to abandon Jonah to the locked-in existence hauntingly elaborated by these parent-authors. There were so many accounts in which the intact mind was successfully recovered, it was hard not to be optimistic. Not all—Josh Greenfeld admits, at the end of the first of three memoirs about his son Noah, that "for all of our hopes and dreams, [we] are still fattening up our children for the inevitable institutional kill. For that is the setting they seemed destined for."[15] And Hughes similarly acknowledges "how far Walker is from where we hoped he'd be by age fifteen."[16]

But those unhappy endings were rare. Besides, Jonah's intelligence had been evident his entire life. When he was fifteen months old, he loved to crawl across the pool table and line up the balls in order from 1 to 15, and he somehow learned to read and write before he could talk—a skill we only discovered when he started printing the titles of *Sesame Street* videos in chalk on the driveway. As he developed some verbal language—rough and garbled at the beginning, never easy for strangers to comprehend—he would occasionally resort to spelling if he thought he wasn't being understood, such as the morning he woke me before dawn by pulling on my arm and demanding, "G-E-T-U-P."

Not that there were any guarantees. I knew the autism spectrum encompassed a broad range of presentations, from the odd genius of Asperger's syndrome to the often profound cognitive, functional, and behavioral challenges of autistic disorder. And that was just the picture of autism circa 2003 or so. The diagnostic categories and criteria were different before then and have changed since. Arguably, there is no more unstable diagnosis in all of medicine. Autism has been described as "rare"[17] and now as an "epidemic";[18] it was considered at first a psychiatric disorder closely related to schizophrenia, and is now grouped with developmental disorders like cerebral palsy (CP) and Down syndrome; it originally connoted "good cognitive potentialities,"[19] but today as many as half of autistic children are also intellectually disabled.

Given the wild ride that autism has taken since child psychiatrist Leo Kanner first proposed the "unique syndrome" he called "inborn autistic disturbances of affective contact" in 1943, the pervasiveness and persistence of the intact mind in autism discourse is particularly striking. My exploration takes me into influential literatures in intellectual and developmental disability, psychoanalysis, psychiatry, and disability rights, but my primary archive is autism parent memoirs. Although "often overlooked," as sociologist Allison Carey has argued, these accounts are critical not because of their accuracy or their generalizability (for they might be neither), but because they play a pivotal role in "shap[ing] the public discourse related to disability."[20] This is undoubtedly why scholars are increasingly turning to them as source material, such as historian Marga Vicedo, who published an entire book on autism parent memoirist Clara Claiborne Park, and critical disability theorist Amanda Apgar, who opens her 2023 analysis *The Disabled Child: Memoirs of a Normal Future* with a claim strikingly similar to Carey's: "Parents and their narratives make significant contributions to shaping public perceptions of disability."[21] More broadly, there is strong consensus in the academy that popular narratives have tremendous impact; disability scholars David Mitchell and Sharon Snyder note that "Americans learn perspectives on disability from books and films more than from policies or personal interactions."[22]

Of particular interest to me is how these autism parent memoirs both reflect and challenge prevalent medical and societal attitudes. In the 1960s, when Park was writing, both psychoanalytic thinking and new understandings of CP were consonant with the promise of the intact mind. But even after medical theories of autism sharply diverged in the 1980s, converging instead around biological causes and dim prognoses, parent-authors were not discouraged. The intact mind is just as robust in autism parent memoirs today as it was fifty years ago—as is evidenced by the title of one 2020 example, *I Know You're in There,* by Marcia Hinds.

The key question for me is: Why? What work does the intact mind do for parent-authors, for readers, for the larger world of policymakers and the public?

And this, also, the implied but unspoken obverse: What about the *impaired* mind?

* * *

It turned out that the early skills we considered signs of Jonah's genius were actually evidence of hyperlexia, a precocious ability to decode text, but not necessarily understand it, that is seen in as much as 20% of autistic children.[23] Now, at age twenty-four, Jonah can still read anything (and he can say the alphabet backward as fast as he can say it forward, which is kind of a cool party trick), but he can't follow the story in a simple board book. He can't answer questions that begin with "why" or "how," or engage in reciprocal conversation unless it's heavily scripted.

I'm not sure exactly when I realized that Jonah has no abstract language, and that the things he says and writes— "pink waterslide," "ketchup and French fries," and, over and over, "Aunt Keri," his favorite person—comprehensively reflect what he thinks about. There was no one moment. It was a process of many years, coming to terms with the fact that loving Jonah—just like loving anyone, really—means accepting him as he is, rather than pretending that he's someone he's not.

Among parents, I found many peers—but not among scholars. The Disability Rights Movement (DRM)—as well as its academic arm, Disability Studies—has had a profound influence on how disability is conceptualized. In the 1970s, academics and advocates rejected the assumption that there was anything bad or wrong with physical impairment and argued that disability resulted instead from a societal failure to accommodate different bodies—for example, by providing curb cuts, elevators, sign-language interpreters, and other supports that would vastly increase the accessibility of public spaces.[24] This "social model of disability" catalyzed a demand for changes to the built environment based not on charity or pity, but on the rights of the disabled to enjoy the same opportunities as the nondisabled.[25]

During this period, disability scholar Philip Ferguson has argued, "'Disability' becomes, in effect, a synonym for 'physical disability' in much of the writing about the disability rights movement."[26] The intellectually disabled are later absorbed into the movement—but only those whose stories can be shoehorned into the social model of disability. It's no coincidence that Carrie Buck becomes the face of intellectual disability history in the United States. Of course her involuntary sterilization and the 1927 Supreme Court decision that authorized it represent a landmark case in American eugenic ideology and practice that is of undeniable interest to researchers.[27] But, even more broadly, Buck's story comports perfectly with the claim made by sociologist James Trent in 1994 that "mental retardation is a construction"[28]—a position that, critical disability theorist Madeline Burghardt confirmed almost a quarter of a century later, has become "*de rigeur* in disability scholarship."[29] Buck's impoverished background, her sexual assault, and her illegitimate pregnancy clearly motivated her institutionalization more than any intellectual disability, which was suspiciously established ex post facto. And the real trump card in the social construction argument? Buck's daughter Vivian—the "third generation" in Justice Oliver Wendell Holmes's infamous declaration that "three generations of imbeciles are enough"—qualified for her school's honor roll, before dying at the age of eight.[30]

Examples of the social construction of intellectual disability represent the truly low-hanging fruit of disability history—illustrated most obviously in shifting diagnostic criteria that doubled or halved the population with the stroke of a pen. In 1910, psychologist (and prominent eugenicist) Henry Goddard proposed replacing Isaac Kerlin's 1877 categories of "superior grades . . . orphaned idiots and imbeciles; and lower grades" with a more expansive label of "feeblemindedness" that included idiots and imbeciles and added the new classification of "moron," which increased the percentage of the affected population from 1% to 2%. More than sixty years later, that move was effectively reversed when the American Association on Mental Deficiency revised their own IQ-based definitions from one to two standard deviations below the mean[31]—and that doesn't even factor in the extensive research challenging the descriptive and prognostic utility of these assessments in the first place.[32] I can only assume that it is those caught in this intersectional gray zone, where fate is overdetermined by education, race, gender, and class, that disability researchers Patrick McDonagh, C. F. Goodey, and Tim Stainton were thinking of when they posed the question, "In short, is intellectual disability an impairment at all?" which they then answered, "In the long historical sweep, it is not."[33]

Similar sentiments inform the DRM-affiliated Autism Rights Movement, which launched in 1993 at the International Conference on Autism, when autistic self-advocate Jim Sinclair scolded parents not to "mourn for us" because the tragedy is not autism itself, but the fact that "your world has no place for us to be."[34] Five years later, another self-advocate, Judy Singer, coined the now more popular term "neurodiversity" to describe a new politics to add to the "categories of class/gender/race and . . . augment the insights of the social model of disability."[35]

Lowercase "neurodiversity" is a truism—minds obviously vary tremendously, including a broad range of intellectual, developmental, and psychiatric disorders, and all fully belong to our human community. But "Neurodiversity" with a capital "N" has come to represent a much more specific position: "that instead of viewing this gift [autism] as an error of nature—a puzzle to be solved and eliminated with techniques like prenatal testing and selective abortion—society should regard it as a valuable part of humanity's genetic legacy."[36] The goal of this movement, as identified by the Autistic Self-Advocacy Network (ASAN), is to "celebrat[e] our differences . . . to make sure that everyone gets the accommodations we need . . . [and] to make sure that autistic people are in control of our own lives, and have a say in policies that affect us."[37]

The right of self-determination, for those with the capacity for it, is also uncontroversial. What has caused much strife in the autism community is the claim by some autistic self-advocates that they speak for the entire spectrum, even those whose profound cognitive impairments preclude self-advocacy. In response to parents like me who have repeatedly countered that the Neurodiversity policy agenda—which rejects all disability-specific educational, vocational, or residential settings—doesn't meet the needs of our kids, whose extreme behavioral and/or medical challenges often require intensive, specialized supports, some autistic self-advocates have adopted a new strategy. "THERE IS NO SUCH THING AS SEVERE AUTISM," tweeted John Marble, founder of the San Francisco–based advocacy organization Pivot Diversity, echoing McDonagh, Goodey, and Stainton's dismissal of intellectual disability. "Just as there is no such thing as 'severe homosexuality' or 'severe blackness.' "[38]

That's where we are now: the impaired mind is flatly denied. It doesn't matter that my son has bloodied his own nose and given himself cauliflower ear from a compulsion to hit himself in the head, over which he has no control. Or that he has shoved his favorite things under the baseboards and down the toilet and screamed in frustration when they couldn't be retrieved. Or that he can't cross the street without supervision or be left alone in the house. Ferguson observed this elision a dozen years before Jonah was born: "The exclusion of people with severe retardation from the disability rights movement is not simply an oversight," he wrote. "[It] is also a logical concomitant of the conceptual base."[39]

Reckoning with the impaired mind is not easy. It requires that we rethink our conceptions of agency, of personhood, of citizenship. But insisting that there are only intact minds is worse—a "denial," sociologist Tom Shakespeare writes, "of the pervasive and sometimes devastating impact of autism on both the child and the family."[40] And, increasingly, other scholars from diverse disciplines are following his lead and challenging strong social constructionist depictions of intellectual and developmental disability that assume the intact mind. English professor Mark Osteen argues that "disability scholarship has ignored cognitive, intellectual, or neurological disabilities, thereby excluding the intellectually disabled just as mainstream society has done."[41] Political scientist Stacy Clifford Simplican observes, "Even when they aim to be inclusive, disability scholars and disability rights activists often call upon cognitive norms of autonomy and empowerment that redraw the boundaries of personhood and reify exclusion."[42] And philosopher Eva Feder Kittay elegantly flips the script: "It is not dependency but independence that is a social construct."[43]

* * *

Perhaps this all sounds a bit familiar. Not necessarily the specific phrase "intact mind," but certainly the heavy tilt of autism discourse toward "the cure story"[44] has been well documented. Disabled writer Michael Whelan observes that "most pathographies [illness narratives] follow some variation of the narrative arc of the quest narrative"—which inevitably ends in victory for the hero—and autism narratives are no exception.[45] Bryna Siegel writes, "Americans dwell on myths of autistic geniuses and miraculous recoveries, ignoring the autism most families face."[46] And theologian James Fisher defines the "conversion narrative" as "a record of the quest for a transformed or redeemed self," and argues that "the history of the autism conversion narrative *is* the history of autism in America."[47]

So what does the specific concept of the intact mind add to this literature? While there are obvious overlaps among "recovery," "conversion," "cure," and "intact mind," they are not synonyms: not all memoirs that invoke the intact mind are recovery narratives, and not all recovery narratives feature the intact mind. Robert Hughes's son, for example, remains profoundly disabled at the end of his book, despite the tantalizing glimpses of what Hughes calls "Walker the Regular Kid . . . peeping through the Special Needs shield."[48] On the flip side, other parent-authors describe their children's recovery from autism—such as Annabel Stehli's account of her daughter's transformation through auditory training,[49] or Karyn Seroussi's about how her son was cured by a gluten- and casein-free diet[50]—without ever suggesting that their children's intact minds were there all along, and would have remained trapped without these interventions.

This difference has extraordinarily important political implications. Narratives of healing and even cure still allow space for the impaired mind, since there are obviously many severely autistic children who grow into severely autistic adults, like Jonah. While they don't dwell on this outcome, these discourses are not ideologically incompatible with disability-specific supports—like the autism school that was recommended after Jonah broke a teacher's nose in our district's inclusive kindergarten class, for example. But if even the most seemingly cognitively impaired individuals have minds that are intact, even if completely inaccessible, then the logical conclusion is that they must have the same values, needs, and preferences as the neurotypical and should be served exclusively in the same settings. And this is exactly what has happened: as the intact mind was consolidated over almost half a century of autism parent memoirs, and as skyrocketing incidence rates made autism eclipse Down syndrome as "the paradigmatic developmental disability . . . of the postmodern period,"[51] this assumption has come to inform much practice and policy for individuals with a range of intellectual and developmental disabilities, leading to drastic changes in the options available to people like Jonah.

* * *

Chasing the Intact Mind is divided into two halves that do not need to be read consecutively. The first half offers a historical analysis of the intact mind: Where did it come from? Why has it persisted? Importantly, this idea does not reflect anything biologically true about autism. Instead, as I argue in this section, it emerged largely from psychoanalytic theory as well as new understandings about CP, and was subsequently amplified by decades of parent-authors documenting their fight—successful or not—to access the "normal" child they knew was trapped within the autistic shell.

Chapter 1, "Valuing the Disabled Child," focuses on the prehistory of autism parent memoirs—accounts by parents of children diagnosed with other types of intellectual and developmental disabilities that first appeared in 1950. These parent-authors loved their kids just as much as the parents of autistic children do, but they wrote about them very differently. Not one of these authors suggests that children with Down syndrome, phenylketonuria (PKU), or other forms of congenital intellectual disability really wouldn't be cognitively impaired after all, if only the proper intervention could be found to break through to them. Instead, these parents emphasized the inherent value of children who were not particularly valued by their communities, while challenging eugenic ideologies that stigmatized families by characterizing such impairments as hereditary, manifestations of degenerate stock.

Where the intact mind does become evident is in early memoirs about CP, which also date to this period. By the mid-twentieth century, physicians had discovered that many individuals who were nonverbal and otherwise profoundly physically disabled by CP actually had typical or even gifted intellects. These books, by priming the American public to see the possibility of intelligence even in the absence of its typical signifiers—such as speech or sign language—lay the groundwork for the embrace of the intact mind.

Chapter 2, "Whose Fault Is It?," discusses the influence of psychoanalytic theory on public understanding of autism—a relative newcomer to the psychiatric scene, having first been described in 1943. Originally considered a form of childhood schizophrenia, autism was conceptualized in the same way as other psychiatric conditions at the time: not as an innate disability, but as a reversible consequence of bad parenting—with bad mothers particularly targeted. Clara Claiborne Park wrote the first autism parent memoir, *The Siege,* in 1967 to challenge this narrative. But even as she sharply defended herself and all the other mothers who had been blamed for their children's impairments, she did so in psychoanalytic imagery that reified this framework from that point forward. By describing her daughter's autism as a "solitary citadel," a "fortress" to be "assail[ed]" through an unrelenting but ultimately successful "siege,"[52] Park not only used the exact same architectural metaphors so prevalent in the psychoanalytic literature, but she centered the intact mind in autism discourse, confirming that—with enough persistence, faith, and hard work—the intelligent, desired child could be recovered.

Chapter 3, "Is There a Key?," follows the intact mind into the autism memoir boom of the 1990s and beyond. By this time, psychiatry looked very different: biological psychiatry had eclipsed psychoanalysis, and most autism researchers and clinicians had agreed for the past decade that the disorder was both physiologically based and incurable. Although happy to be acquitted by the medical establishment, parents refused to accept such bleak prognoses—especially ones that were so discordant with their own experiences or breakthroughs they had read about. The intact mind continues to thrive—not only in parent memoirs, but, as I demonstrate in Part II of the book, as a foundational assumption to much policy and practice involving the intellectually and developmentally disabled today.

If you don't need to be convinced of the importance or the contingency of the intact mind in autism discourse, or if you are simply more interested in its contemporary impact, feel free to start with the case studies of

Part II. Chapter 4 focuses on the fight to close 14(c) vocational programs, also known as sheltered workshops, which employ significantly intellectually and developmentally disabled individuals at a subminimum wage. Catalyzing the increasingly successful push to eliminate this model is the insistence by Neurodiversity proponents and Disability Rights advocates more generally that everyone is capable of holding competitive, minimum-wage employment if the appropriate supports are provided. Not only is this assertion not supported by any data, but the few studies that have tracked outcomes in states following the elimination of 14(c) have found that most participants end up sitting at home, because their significant cognitive impairments and dangerous behaviors preclude their participation in integrated employment.

The second case study (Chapter 5) analyzes the push to replace legal guardianship with a more casual model, known as Supported Decision Making (SDM), that empowers the cognitively impaired to choose their own informal advisors. However, unlike guardianship—which involves court approval and oversight—SDM requires no external supervision or other protective measures. There is no recourse for intellectually disabled people who are convinced by their "friends" to invest in sketchy business enterprises or to forgo necessary medical procedures. Advanced most prominently by the United Nations, SDM advocacy is predicated on the explicit claim that all people with autism or other forms of intellectual and developmental disability are capable of making their own choices—regarding housing, direct care staff, medical procedures, and other complex and consequential decisions—no matter how severe their cognitive impairments.

Finally, in Chapter 6, I turn to facilitated communication (FC), a controversial practice in which a nondisabled "facilitator" helps a profoundly intellectually disabled and minimally or completely nonverbal "user" to communicate via a letterboard through physical contact of some kind: holding the letterboard, or supporting the user at the wrist, elbow, or shoulder. Although three decades of controlled studies have repeatedly proved that the output of these interactions is directed by the facilitators, not the users, interest in these techniques is exploding, as practitioners promise to help desperate parents unlock the intact minds within their severely autistic children.

These cases all pit advocates, family members, and providers who assume the intact mind and privilege the autonomy they celebrate as a fundamental human right against those who, like bioethicist Paul Appelbaum, defend a different right—that of incapacitated individuals "to protection from the consequences of their conditions."[53] Missing from these debates, however, is any explicit engagement with the intact mind. It is my hope that foregrounding this concept—examining its origins, interrogating its stakeholders, and articulating both its assumptions and implications—will ultimately make space not only for the impaired mind, but also for the networks of interdependence that center new frameworks of care.

PART I
THE HISTORY OF THE INTACT MIND

1

Valuing the Disabled Child

The Emergence of Disability Memoirs, 1950–1956

Before there were autism parent memoirs, there were parent memoirs about children with other forms of intellectual and developmental disability. Although these early exemplars followed a much different trajectory than most of the autism parent memoirs that would follow, it's worth examining them in some detail—not only to untangle the origins of the intact mind, but to show that this concept was neither inevitable, nor the only possible response to significant cognitive impairment.

The first parent memoir about intellectual disability was Pearl Buck's *The Child Who Never Grew*. It was published in 1950, when Buck's daughter Carol was thirty years old, but if her opening line was any indication, it represented a project she had been struggling with for decades: "I have been a long time making up my mind to write this story."[1] Later, Buck would learn that Carol suffered from what we now know as phenylketonuria (PKU), an inability to metabolize the amino acid phenylalanine for which all infants are now routinely screened, as the symptoms—including cognitive impairment, seizures, eczema, and behavioral challenges—can be prevented through dietary adjustments. But in 1924, all Buck knew was that her four-year-old daughter's "mind had stopped growing."[2] This short account follows Buck from China, where she lived most of her life, to the United States. Desperate for answers, she bounced from doctor to doctor, until a staff member at the Mayo Clinic—notably not the psychologist who had just given her an ambiguous, indecisive report—finally spoke plainly: "[Carol] will never be able to speak properly. She will never be able to read and write, she will never be more than about four years old, at best. Prepare yourself, madame!"[3]

Buck and Carol returned to China, but by 1929 they were back in the United States in search of an institutional placement. Buck credits a terrifying incident for catalyzing this decision, in which the family (by this point, she and her then-husband John had adopted a daughter) was forced to hide with neighbors while Communist soldiers attacked foreigners; also influential was the growing realization that Carol would always be ostracized in their expat community. Part III of Buck's memoir describes the methodical process by which she selected the Vineland Training School in New Jersey, where Carol lived until her death in 1992.

Buck kept Carol a secret from the public for more than twenty years before writing *The Child Who Never Grew.*[4] But she ultimately broke her silence because, she said, she wanted "my child's life to be of use in her generation."[5] On a purely practical level, she advises other parents of intellectually disabled children: how to deal with grief ("There must be acceptance and the knowledge that sorrow fully accepted brings its own gifts. . . . It can be transmuted into wisdom"[6]); how to evaluate an institution (down to the need for a "self-perpetuating board of trustees"[7]); how to remain involved in their children's lives post-institutionalization ("Do not think that secret bribes or tips will protect your child from a bad attendant"[8]).

More broadly, however, Buck appeals to a public that she knows finds little value in the intellectually disabled. She adopts a two-pronged strategy in this campaign: first, she describes how parenting Carol made her a better person: "My helpless child has taught me so much. She has taught me patience, above all else." This instrumental view of the disabled, emphasizing their positive impact on those around them, becomes a common theme in disability parent memoirs going forward—including one that appeared three years after Buck's, written by one of the most beloved personalities in the country.

In 1953, Dale Evans Rogers—wife of cowboy Roy Rogers—published a book about the couple's daughter Robin, who had Down syndrome. This revelation was news to the Rogers' millions of fans, as—like Buck—they had kept Robin's condition a secret "from all but their families and close friends," Maxine Garrison, an assistant publicity director for Roy Rogers Enterprises, wrote in her own book about those years. "The ever-inquiring reporters and photographers were necessarily told that Robin's delicate heart condition made visitors and pictures impossible."[9]

It's hard to characterize Evans Rogers's account as a memoir, exactly—*Angel Unaware* is narrated in the first person by Robin herself, who meets God in heaven immediately following her death from mumps encephalitis at the age of two and tells him about her adventures "Down There." In the context of the intact mind, it's tempting to interpret the maturity of Robin's narrative voice as an early claim by Evans Rogers about her daughter's inner capacity. But *Angel Unaware* isn't about accuracy—no typical two-year-old speaks like the narrator, never mind a two-year-old with a developmental disability. More accurately, it reflects traditional Christian doctrine that believers are healed of all illness and impairment upon reaching the kingdom of heaven; as Robin tells God on the first page, "I'm perfectly all right, now that I'm rid of that lump of hindering clay."[10]

There's not much in this short volume of what we would call today the "lived experience" of disability; at the end we know as little about the flesh-and-blood Robin as we did at the start, when the narrator sets up what is to follow as an account of her "earthly mission." Practically, she celebrates her parents' commitment to use their fame and wealth to help children with intellectual disabilities. But it's clear that her primary purpose was to bring her family closer to God. One of Roy Rogers's first reactions to his daughter's birth, Robin reports, was to "read his Bible as though he had never seen it before. And he prayed, more and more often. . . . A new Roy Rogers was being born."[11] Her mother experienced a similar awakening; Robin tells God, "I heard Mommy say one day that she was coming to believe that the only important thing in this world was a person's relationship to God and his faith in Jesus Christ." Crucially, Evans Rogers emphasizes through her narrator, Robin deserves all the credit for her parents' transformation: "[Mommy] said she was actually grateful to you for sending me in my handicapped condition, because I had made her walk closer to you."[12] And it wasn't just her parents—Robin's influence extended to her half-siblings, who became "more and more unselfish and [did] more and more for people who were weaker than they were," as well as the family doctor, who decided to go to "theological school to equip himself, spiritually, so that he could be of more help to the parents of other problem babies like me."[13]

But even more groundbreaking and impactful was the second prong in Buck's strategy, which was also adopted by Evans Rogers. Beyond their daughters' influence on others, these women celebrated an intrinsic value comparable to nondisabled children—who, sociologist Viviana Zelizer has argued, had become "sacralized" during the long Progressive Era. By the 1930s, education had been expanded, playgrounds were built, and child labor was largely abolished, stripping children of the economic value they had held in the eighteenth century—particularly for rural parents who conceived of them as future farmhands—and shifting them to "a special and separate world, regulated by affection and education, not work or profit."[14] John Gunther's enormously popular 1949 account of the passing of his seventeen-year-old son Johnny from a brain tumor perfectly illustrates this new understanding of children's worth. His death represented a tremendous loss—not of labor, or economic support in his parents' old age, but of an irreplaceable individual celebrated for his "sweetness, his remarkable goodness and pure, ineffable niceness."[15]

But those weren't all, or even the most important, of Johnny's attributes. Bound for Harvard before his illness, and so brilliant and determined he completed over fifty chemistry experiments while convalescing at home following multiple surgeries, x-ray treatment, and other interventions, Gunther notes the unbearable irony that his son was "afflicted in that part of him which was his best, the brain."[16] This was what made Buck's and Evans Rogers's books so revolutionary: their insistence that their cognitively impaired daughters deserved to have their stories told as well, that they were equally—to use Zelizer's term—as "priceless" as an intellectual powerhouse like Johnny Gunther. "Mind is not all of the human creature," Buck gently reminds us. "All people are equal in their humanity and . . . all have the same human rights. None is to be considered less, as a human being, than any other, and each must be given his place and safety in the world."[17] Agreed Evans Rogers, with a more religious spin, "There are many mansions, or 'rooms,' in [God's] earthly house. . . . A room for everyone and something for them to do in that room for [God]."[18]

This represented a truly transgressive claim in the mid-twentieth century. Much more common was rhetoric such as that with which anthropologist Walter Goldschmidt introduced his 1967 study on the intellectually disabled: "Of all the attributes of man, mind is the quintessence; to be found wanting in mental capacity—in general intellectual competence—is the most devastating of all possible stigmata."[19] As late as 1984, historians Peter Tyor and Leland Bell were describing "mental deficiency" as "the most profound disability, a crippling handicap which can be ameliorated but never cured. Historically, it has carried a mark of shame, identifying the afflicted as a subhuman creature, a vegetable, or a blob of flesh." Echoing sociologist Erving Goffman's classic analysis on stigma, particularly how it spreads to family and friends, Tyor and Bell add, "Tortured and dismayed by this reality, parents and relatives of the retarded have been overwhelmed with feelings of guilt, failure, and futility, and they, too, suffer social stigmatization."[20]

This guilt arose from centuries of blaming parents for the intellectual disabilities of their children. Concerns with the hereditability of mental abnormality date back to 1621, when Oxford fellow Robert Burton argued that melancholy (known as depression today) was "an hereditary disease" that parents could pass down to their children "by Propagation."[21] Two centuries later, French psychiatrist Bénédict Morel introduced the concept of degeneration in 1857 to explain how "a deteriorating environment could lead the species to degenerate—physically, intellectually, and morally."[22] This resulted in a host of undesirable sequelae, including idiocy, alcoholism, poverty, insanity, inbreeding, and others.

The most prominent American degenerationist, Richard Dugdale, actually emphasized the importance of environmental factors, considering them equally if not more important than heredity. In his landmark family history *The Jukes: A Study in Crime, Pauperism, Disease and Heredity*, published in 1877, Dugdale traced the outcomes of hundreds of members of one poor, rural New York family (which, he acknowledged, was actually a composite of dozens of families). Many of his subjects had ended up in jail—but not all of them. Dugdale suggested that an inborn predisposition to "harlotry," for example, could be trumped by a change in situation, such as an early marriage. "Where the environment changes in youth the characteristics of heredity may be measurably altered," he pronounced.[23] But that's not what his contemporaries heard. Inflamed with the rhetoric of Charles Darwin and later validated by the rediscovery of Mendel's laws of heredity in 1900, social Darwinists like Francis Galton and Charles Davenport proclaimed that "biology was destiny"[24]—a conviction Henry Goddard was able to prove in 1912 by applying Dugdale's method of pedigree studies to the perfect natural experiment: the Kallikak family, a pseudonym Goddard created by combining the Greek words for beauty (*kallos*) and bad (*kakos*).

Goddard's ground zero was Martin Kallikak, Sr., who had a dalliance with a "feeble-minded" tavern girl during the Revolutionary War and fathered an illegitimate son. After the War, Martin Sr. married a "respectable girl of good family." Each line produced almost five hundred descendants, who turned out pretty much how a good degenerationist would predict: on the tavern girl's side, the family was plagued by feeblemindedness, alcoholism, epilepsy, prostitution, and licentiousness. On the other side, in stark contrast, were "descendants of colonial governors, signers of the Declaration of Independence, soldiers and even the founders of a great university. . . . Half a dozen towns in New Jersey are named from the families into which Martin's descendants have married."[25] Goddard published his study accompanied by neat charts demonstrating to his satisfaction that feeblemindedness was a "unit character" subject to the same predictable laws of inheritance Mendel had demonstrated in his pea plants and that had already been shown to apply to some traits in humans, like hair color and albinism.

Historians Steven Noll and James Trent describe *The Kallikak Family* as "possibly the most influential book in the history of mental retardation in America."[26] By 1939, it had been reprinted a dozen times and was cited in the most prominent eugenic debates both at home and abroad—it was submitted as evidence in the 1927 Supreme Court case *Buck v. Bell*, which authorized the involuntary sterilization of the intellectually disabled, and was translated into German in 1933, the same year the "Law for Prevention of Offspring with Hereditary Defects Act" was passed.[27]

But by then, American scientific and medical interest in eugenics had waned. It had become increasingly evident that feeblemindedness and other associated markers of degeneration did not follow Mendel's dominant/recessive hereditary patterns. The conflation of eugenics with Nazi atrocities finalized the divorce, and after World War II, American researchers and clinicians largely changed the official line on intellectual disability. "Most cases of extreme retardation are not the result of heredity," psychologist Samuel Kirk and colleagues assured parents in *You and Your Retarded Child: A Manual for Parents of Retarded Children.*[28] Agreed pediatrician Abraham Levinson in another guidebook, "There is not a single family that has not suffered some deviation from the normal at one time or another."[29] But the public was still largely unconvinced. Despite these affirmations from prominent physicians, historian Katherine Castles argues, "mental retardation was still often viewed as part of a more general, genetically based social deviance that might reveal the 'bad stock' of the entire family."[30]

This is undoubtedly why Buck and Evans Rogers so explicitly and decisively reject the "bad stock" assumption. In *Angel Unaware*, Robin recounts a conversation her mother had with a prominent doctor: "He told Mommy that this affliction was no respecter of persons, that it hits anywhere, anytime. One of his friends, a top baby doctor, had a baby just like me."[31] Buck took a more scientific tack, reporting, "Almost one person in every hundred is or will be mentally retarded, and of these the majority are retarded from non-inherited causes. The old stigma of 'something in the family' is all too often unjust." Later, she reminds readers that "there was nothing in my family to make me fear that my child might be one of those who do not grow. Indeed, I was fortunate in my own ancestry on both sides. My father's family was distinguished for achievement in languages and letters, and my mother's family was a cultivated one."[32]

It took a tremendous amount of social capital to successfully challenge such an entrenched narrative—and that's what Buck and Evans Rogers had, along with a not insignificant amount of the traditional kind of capital (a fact that did not go unnoticed by some readers, including Lucille Stout, who in 1959 published a memoir about her own daughter with Down syndrome that included one of the few critiques of *Angel Unaware* I have found: "I was disappointed in the story of Robin Rogers. It left me untouched and unhelped. Where I had not been able to provide even a separate room for my child, that family could build a separate house and staff it for their child. Their prestige was such that they did not have to worry about social stigma"[33]). Both Buck and Evans Rogers were hugely famous when their memoirs were published: Buck, the popular author of *The Good Earth*, had already been awarded both the Pulitzer and Nobel prizes (in 1932 and 1938, respectively), and Evans Rogers and her husband Roy "were the most recognized movie and television couple in America, and maybe, in the world."[34]

Disability scholar Stuart Murray argues that such celebrities have more freedom to tackle sensitive subjects because their celebrity "pushes what otherwise can be an unsettling topic into the realm of star biography" and thus "blunts the edge of a subject that a majority audience might find troubling."[35] Historian and physician Barron Lerner focuses less on the sanitizing effect of celebrity illness narratives than their unique power to impact public perception and policy. One of Lerner's case studies features baseball player Jimmy Piersall, who described his experience with bipolar disorder in an autobiography contemporaneous with *The Child Who Never Grew* and *Angel Unaware*—the first time, according to wife Mary Piersall, "anyone in the public eye had ever openly identified himself as a former mental patient."[36]

Fear Strikes Out, published in 1955, was a tremendous commercial success, selling hundreds of thousands of copies. "The topic of mental illness in a famous person, formerly seen as taboo," Lerner noted, "had become compelling."[37] Buck and Evans Rogers had the same impact for intellectual disability. Both books were excerpted or profiled in popular magazines, including *Readers' Digest* and *Time*, and *Angel Unaware* sold the third-most copies of any title published in 1953, behind the *Revised Standard Version of the Bible* and *The Power of Positive Thinking*.[38] And both were credited with changing the public's attitude toward cognitive impairment: Kirk and his colleagues introduced their 1955 guidebook by celebrating "this recent change in attitude toward mental retardation" which was "the result of frank expressions by parents . . . . Pearl Buck, Dale Evans Rogers and many others have written about their experiences."[39]

No doubt, the Buck and Evans Rogers books received the most attention at the time and have consumed the bulk of the historiographical oxygen since. But a consideration of the *third* most prominent parent disability memoir of the period offers useful insight into the importance of status in tackling what was—as Evans Rogers acknowledged in a preface to the 1981 edition of *Angel Unaware*—a "subject no other publisher would touch with a ten-foot pole."[40]

John P. Frank's *My Son's Story* was published right between *Angel* and *The Child Who Never Grew*. Frank wasn't famous then, but he would be, at least in legal circles. He was a lawyer who would go on to shape the argument in *Brown v. Board of Education*, as well as to represent Ernesto Miranda in the Supreme Court case that led to the establishment of the Miranda warning. But in 1952, he was just a Yale law professor—impressive, no doubt, but maybe not quite impressive enough. How else to explain the multiple cameos by Supreme

Court Justices in *My Son's Story*, giants Frank knew from his days as a law clerk for Justice Hugo Black a decade earlier? Even more important than this name-dropping is the work these celebrities do: the important themes in Frank's memoir are notably articulated not in his own voice, but in letters he quotes from the Justices. In support of the decision to institutionalize his son John Peter, who had been diagnosed with cortical atrophy, at eighteen months, Frank cites a cautionary tale from Justice Black: "'A cousin of mine permitted a child that was mentally helpless to be in the home with other children. It cast a blight over the lives of the parents and the children.'" And Justice Wiley Rutledge weighs in on the assumed guilt of the parents, writing, "'Of course neither [Frank's wife Lorraine] nor anyone else should feel the least tinge of a sense of shame about the matter. . . . The thing could happen to anyone at any time and it is a matter beyond any possible individual control.'"[41]

It worked: *My Son's Story*, like *The Child Who Never Grew* before it, "received widespread public attention"; it was featured in *Time* and excerpted by *Readers' Digest*,[42] and it was celebrated more than fifteen years later as "one of the earliest and best books by a parent of a retarded child" and "a great human document."[43] By deploying their status (both real and vicarious), Buck, Frank, and Evans Rogers opened the door to a flood of parent disability memoirs—not by celebrities, but by civilian parents (and occasionally siblings)—that still hasn't stopped. The books that came out over the next decade were similarly concerned with absolving parents of any responsibility for their children's intellectual disabilities: in *Betty Lee*, published in 1954, Charlotte D. Tucker reminds us that "handicapped children . . . are all around us. Few families escape. . . . Handicaps appear without respect to persons, place, or time; they reach into every state of society."[44] Dorothy Garst Murray included an exonerating letter from her cousin, who worked at the Mayo Clinic, in her 1956 memoir, *This Is Stevie's Story*: "'Why should you feel shame for a biological accident? And your other clearly superior children are all the proof needed that it is a biological accident.'"[45] Five years later, Carvel Lee opened her memoir with a veritable pedigree to prove that her sister Jeanie's cognitive impairments were not inherited. "Both Mother and Dad were of high intelligence," Lee reports. "Both grandfathers had been ministers, and their capable wives had shared their lives of service. Uncles and aunts we had in abundance, but none of them had shown symptoms of mental deficiency."[46]

Starting in the mid-1960s, however, parents seemingly no longer felt the need to make such claims. New research was beginning to unravel the physiological causes of—and sometimes, even treatments for—the most common intellectual disabilities. In 1954, a team of doctors in the United Kingdom announced that a diet low in the amino acid phenylalanine prevented the cognitive impairments that developed otherwise in children with PKU, the metabolic disorder suffered by Carol Buck.[47] And in 1959, French physician Jérôme Lejeune found the genetic cause of Down syndrome: an extra copy of the twenty-first chromosome. Older theories that had implicated the mother's alcoholism, syphilis, and even "rebellion against the marriage"[48] now sounded hopelessly outdated. In his 1964 history of intellectual disability, prominent child psychiatrist and originator of the autism diagnosis Leo Kanner dismissed decades of eugenic targeting of the cognitively impaired population as "emotionally charged blasts"—noting, in a cavalier style that was typical for him, "It did not seem to occur to the preachers of gloom that civilization was indeed in grave danger but that the danger did not come from the mental defectives. . . . The one man Hitler, who probably would not have come out too badly in terms of the Binet-Simon scale, did more damage than all the mental defectives since the beginning of history."[49]

Instead of defending themselves, parents of children with Down syndrome and other forms of significant cognitive impairments typically emphasized one of Buck's and Evans Rogers's other themes: the value of the intellectually disabled to their families and greater communities. Often this assumed a religious valence similar to *Angel Unaware*, as in Sophia Gant's 1957 memoir *"One of Those": The Progress of a Mongoloid Child*, in which she remembers, "I wondered why Peter wasn't healed instantly, but I know God wanted to teach this family to trust Him fully and to learn more of His word. . . . The more I prayed the better [Peter] looked; the less I prayed the worse he looked."[50] In his 1965 account, *Sunshine: A Slow Miracle*, author B. R. Schmalzreid reflects, "It became evident to me that through my baby my faith had grown stronger, my knowledge and understanding of God fuller, and my desire to requite His love more intense," confirming his wife's initial reaction to the birth of their daughter with Down syndrome: " 'This baby may be our means of getting to heaven.' "[51] And three years later, J. Norman Heard affirmed, "I became convinced years ago that God allowed our children to be mentally retarded in order to show us our purpose in life. It has given us the satisfaction of helping people, once regarded as lifetime dregs of society, to become useful citizens. We hope it has made us better Christians for, certainly, we have had the opportunity to take up the cross and follow Him."[52]

But more secular claims were advanced as well—including in another book by Pearl Buck published fifteen years after *The Child Who Never Grew.* The purpose of this second volume is foregrounded right in the title: *The Gifts They Bring: Our Debt to the Mentally Retarded.* Mused Buck, after more than a decade of advocating for families of intellectually disabled kids, "The entire focus of our attention has been on *what we could do for the retarded*, not on what they do for us," a list she spends the rest of the book compiling. Some of those gifts—such as "the use of retarded children in several outstanding medically oriented projects" like the polio vaccine experiments at Pennsylvania's Polk State School—are for obvious reasons not celebrated in later memoirs, but many are, including lessons on "the value of able leadership," "a clearer understanding of justice," "the intangible quality of love," and "patience and consideration."[53]

This theme has had extraordinary staying power (although, occasionally, you do find pushback against the idea that the disabled should be defined in terms of their value to the nondisabled[54]), connecting accounts by Buck and her contemporaries not only to narratives that closely followed theirs, but also to much more recent projects. In 1968, for example, Nancy Roberts elucidated the lessons she learned from her son David, who had Down syndrome, including "patience, courage to go on, a humility which shatters false pride, and inner questioning of the status quo. . . . The society in which we live could become not only a safer but a kinder environment, an environment more suitable to the growth potential of *all* its people."[55] Thirty years later, Martha Beck—also the mother of a child with Down syndrome—observed, in the bestseller *Expecting Adam*, "Living with Adam, loving Adam, has taught me a lot about the truth. He has taught me to look at things in themselves, not at the value a brutal and often senseless world assigns to them."[56] And Vicki Forman, in her 2009 memoir about her multiply disabled son, delivered at twenty-three weeks, reflected, "I've been given an opportunity: to look at fear, forgive myself, learn how to love (myself, others, my son, no matter how imperfect he may be). . . . It's what I do in the face of this experience that matters."[57]

Critically, however, none of these memoirs of Down syndrome, PKU, or congenital intellectual disability, from the 1950s to the present, employs in any way the narrative of the intact mind. This is not to say that there is no possibility for improvement: Charlotte Tucker notes that "capacities which do exist may be developed and through educational and vocational training may give to [the child] a more satisfactory way of life."[58] And even traditional academic skills are not out of the question—Sophia Gant reports that, through homeschooling, she and her son Peter "covered eight grades in about ten years. . . . Reading, writing, spelling, geography, history, health, English, grammar, composition and French were some of his subjects."[59]

But these modest gains were not at all intended to suggest hope for recovery—which is explicitly articulated in many of these memoirs as a delusion with dangerous consequences. B. R. Schmalzried "remembered the doctor saying how futile it would be to rush into the hallowed halls of specialists in a frantic search for a cure."[60] Tucker's father told her about a friend of his who refused to accept his child's impairments, which " 'not only wrecked him financially, for he not only searched in this country but abroad, but it wrecked his entire life, searching to no avail, for, he said, if there is a serious brain injury at birth it cannot be corrected.' "[61] And John Frank recounts a conversation he had with a doctor when his son John Peter was a year old:

> You may start shopping from doctor to doctor, in hopes of a medical miracle. Don't. . . . I have seen tragedy after tragedy with parents who would not, could not believe the truth. I must warn you that there are charlatans in our profession still, men who will promise miracles at high prices. I know a family that has a child who is a Mongolian idiot. They have traveled over the United States and Europe looking for a cure. They have spent far over ten thousand dollars on medical bills. The child is a Mongolian idiot still.[62]

* * *

But the intact mind is central to one subset of disability memoirs: narratives of cerebral palsy. Doctors had long assumed that patients with the most severe symptoms—including paralysis and the inability to speak—were profoundly cognitively impaired, and such children were frequently abandoned to custodial care in institutions. Because no definitive history of this condition has been written, it's hard to tell exactly when this belief began to be questioned. In his 1952 textbook, *Developmental Disorders of Mentation and Cerebral Palsies*, psychiatrist Clemens Benda reports, as if it is a recent development, "The discovery that children with cerebral palsy frequently are of high intelligence, and that their motor disorder is likely to obscure their mental capabilities, has given a great impetus to the development of cerebral palsy programs."[63] Certainly Marie Killilea encountered a much different attitude in the early 1940s, as she describes in her bestselling 1952 memoir *Karen*: by the time her daughter (who was born in 1941) was three and a half years old, she had seen "twenty-three doctors in two and a half years. We've been all over the country. They all tell us the case is hopeless—that a person with cerebral palsy has no mentality." One doctor recommends that she "take your child to an institution and leave her and forget you ever had her"; another speaks more cruelly (and inaccurately, if Buck's account of the inclusive Chinese attitude toward children of all abilities is given any weight): " 'In China, they have the answer . . . they take such children up on top of a mountain and leave them.' "[64]

Killilea refuses to accept these assessments and does, ironically, exactly what Charlotte Tucker's father warned her not to do. Only

Killilea eventually does find a doctor who confirms what she already knew: "'There is no question that [Karen] is mentally very alert. Normal IQ or higher.'"[65] The rest of the book recounts not only Karen's physical and academic progress, but Killilea's increasing involvement in parent advocacy, including the launch of the United Cerebral Palsy Association in 1948. Invited to speak with local parents groups all across the country, Killilea was well positioned to assess the mid-century cerebral palsy scene, which she described as "an oft-reiterated report of incorrect diagnosis, faulty prognosis, children growing up confined to bed, ninety-nine out of a hundred receiving no treatment or education, an appreciable number improperly confined to mental institutions because they could not be taken care of at home, others hidden in attics." Greatly troubled by this vision, she laments to her husband, "Think of the loneliness and frustration of so many cerebral palsied, living behind a wall of silence because their speech is unintelligible or they have none at all. Or those hidden and buried in homes or institutions."[66]

Even more poignant were autobiographies by those very "cerebral palsied," which document the tremendous effort to prove the often brilliant intellects inside profoundly uncooperative bodies. In 1941, Earl Carlson published his memoir *Born That Way* about how he graduated from Yale Medical School "despite my inability to walk, my aimlessly jerking arms, and my speech difficulties."[67] And Irish painter and writer Christy Brown's famous memoir *My Left Foot* was released in 1954. Completely nonverbal and only able to control one limb, Brown "was lonely, imprisoned in a world of my own, unable to communicate with others, cut off, separated from them as though a glass wall stood between my existence and theirs," before he learned how to write with chalk with his left foot.[68]

Later narratives of cerebral palsy would diverge on this question: sometimes there was an intact mind, sometimes there wasn't. Joey Deacon—who was born more than a decade before Brown but whose autobiography didn't appear until 1974—describes how his uncontrollable limbs and garbled speech left him unable to communicate before a friend at St. Lawrence's Hospital in England, where both men lived, became his translator. Deacon concludes *Joey: An Unforgettable Story of Human Courage* with a note of gratitude for Ernie: "'I'm just coming up to my fifty-third year. Half of those were silent, half were not, thanks to you. You gave me the chance to talk to the outside world.'"[69] Ruth Sienkiewicz-Mercer's 1989 autobiography *I Raise My Eyes to Say Yes* paints a very similar story of someone who "could not walk, talk, or feed myself" and who was evaluated by a psychologist to have "a mental age of four months" but who was in fact "mentally sharp."[70]

In contrast, Nicola Schaefer is never able to answer the question she poses in the title of her 1978 memoir about her daughter Catherine, who has cerebral palsy, *Does She Know She's There?* The closest she comes is in an update to the first edition, published more than twenty years later: "How Catherine's mind works, what her thought processes are, remain a mystery to me."[71] And Helene Brown opens *Yesterday's Child* with a curt assessment of her daughter Karen, who, at twenty, is "cerebral palsied, mentally retarded, and deaf" and who, by that point, had spent almost half her life in residential schools learning activities of daily living like dressing and feeding herself. Interestingly, Karen's physical disabilities were significantly less involved than those of Deacon or Sienkiewicz-Mercer; Brown describes "a perfect-looking baby with a pretty body [who] had no physical deformity that I could see" who grows into a lovely young woman with "gleaming teeth, shining hair, aquamarine eyes edged with thick dark lashes" who learns to walk and communicate with a basic sign language.[72]

The takeaway from these very diverse accounts? Appearances could not be trusted—not when there was so much at stake: agency, opportunity, even personhood. But, in the absence of independent communication, how could you tell? A fascinating part of both Deacon's and Sienkiewicz-Mercer's memoirs grapples with the labor required to demonstrate the intact mind, describing in detail their writing processes, which required the aid of collaborators. Deacon's speech was only intelligible to one friend, Ernie. But Ernie couldn't read or write, so he repeated Deacon's words to a second friend, Michael. After the transcript was edited by the staff to correct spelling and grammatical errors, Deacon read the entire text out loud, letter by letter (interpreted by Ernie) to a third friend, Tom—who, although illiterate, was able to peck out the letters on a typewriter. Steven Kaplan, credited as Sienkiewicz-Mercer's coauthor, depicts a methodology only slightly less arduous: "Ruth can neither hold the boards nor point to her chosen words or phrases. The listener must position the boards in front of her; using her facial expressions, Ruth then selects the appropriate board. She guides her listener to the desired section of that board either by looking at it or by answering yes-or-no questions as to location with her face. She pinpoints the exact word or phrase in the same fashion." At first, Kaplan recounts, he worried whether "the written product accurately represented her commentary or unwittingly embodied too many of my own projections." But after working with Sienkiewicz-Mercer for months, he realized that "she never willingly permits [me] to misconstrue the message."[73]

Autism parent memoirs, to which I turn in the next chapter, borrow from both these literatures. Like Buck, Evans Rogers, and their near contemporaries, parents of autistic children faced what became a pervasive, often quite hostile accusation that they were responsible for their children's impairments. Their blame, however, was not cast in terms of heredity or degeneration. Even as the pediatricians, neurologists, and asylum superintendents who assumed the care of the intellectually disabled let parents off the etiological hook, child psychiatrists offered explanations for their own patients' perplexing symptoms that were firmly grounded in Freudian assumptions about the importance of the mother-infant relationship to the development of a normal psyche. This proved, for parents, to be a double-edged sword: as devastating as it was to think that they might have somehow caused their children's autism, it also provided hope that, with enough commitment and expert guidance, the intact mind could be recovered.

2

Whose Fault Is It?

Psychoanalysis and the First Autism Parent Memoirs, 1941–1976

Although Leo Kanner published his seminal paper introducing the world to his new diagnosis—provisionally called "autistic disturbances of affective contact," later shortened to "infantile autism"—in 1943, the first autism parent memoir wouldn't appear for another twenty-four years.[1] What took so long? As discussed in the previous chapter, the success of books by "somebodies" Pearl Buck and Dale Evans Rogers opened the door to a wave of "nobody memoirs"[2]—i.e., accounts by non-celebrity parents about their intellectually disabled children. Why didn't any parents of autistic kids follow suit until Clara Claiborne Park published *The Siege* in 1967?

One factor may have been the small number of parents whose children initially received the autism diagnosis. But although Kanner did believe that his new syndrome was rare, reporting in 1958 that he had only diagnosed about 150 children over the past two decades,[3] Dutch psychiatrist D. A. van Krevelen was already "impatient with the confused and confusing use of the term infantile autism as a slogan, indiscriminately applied, with cavalier abandonment of the [diagnostic] criteria."[4] So maybe it wasn't about the lack of autism parents; maybe instead it was about their unwillingness to speak up, to challenge a merciless societal discourse that originated in psychoanalytic theory and was embraced by the popular media. Stuart Murray muses, "It is difficult to imagine how challenging it must have been to be the parent of an autistic child in, say, 1960, even though we know there must have been many of them. . . . The full weight of medical knowledge would have made it very clear where the blame lay."[5]

As mentioned in the Introduction, the classification of autism as a disorder has changed significantly since the 1940s. Today, autism spectrum disorder (ASD) is considered a developmental disability, which the Centers for Disease Control and Prevention (CDC) define as a condition "due to an impairment in physical, learning, language, or behavior areas [that] . . . begin[s] during the developmental period, may impact day-to-day functioning, and usually last[s] throughout a person's lifetime."[6] This groups ASD with spina bifida, attention deficit hyperactivity disorder (ADHD), cerebral palsy, and Down syndrome.

But autism was conceptualized by Kanner very differently, as a psychiatric condition: in his first paper on the disorder, he was careful to note that "even though most of these children were at one time or another looked upon as feebleminded, they are all unquestionably endowed with good *cognitive potentialities*,"[7] and by 1949 he was explicitly proposing that "early infantile autism may therefore be looked upon as the earliest possible manifestation of childhood schizophrenia."[8] This difference—between mental illness and intellectual disability—has been observed since the thirteenth century,[9] but its importance has varied tremendously since then. In the nineteenth century, these conditions were considered related, both by psychiatrists like Charles Mercier, who argued that "in idiocy and weakness of mind, the process of development has not been carried *far enough*; while in insanity, the process has been carried far enough, but has diverged into the *wrong direction*,"[10] and by degenerationists like Bénédict Morel, who simply considered them both examples of the many unfortunate outcomes of bad breeding. And although the two could generally be distinguished—most notably by the fact that mental illness was considered transient, while intellectual disability was permanent—"between these groups," Mercier advised, "no exact line of demarcation can be drawn."[11] As physician William Ireland wondered in 1898, "Why, for example, should there be such a great preponderance of idiots in Austria and Hungary, whereas in Sweden, Denmark, and Belgium there is such a preponderance of the insane?"[12]

Much more recently, disability scholars have taken a similarly inclusive approach. Writing in 2003, Cynthia Lewiecki-Wilson groups these conditions under the rubric of "mental disabilities," a move she justifies by pointing out that both mental illness and intellectual disability challenge traditional definitions of selfhood that rely on agency and language.[13] Margaret Price agrees, arguing for a coalition of advocacy united by the belief, whether or not it is physiologically true, "that one's disability is located in one's mind."[14] Gil Eyal and colleagues locate the disruption of this border with autism itself, which they argue "serve[s] as the hinge connecting the two, mental illness and mental retardation."[15]

But this fuzzy boundary crystallized, for the middle decades of the twentieth century, into an impenetrable wall built on the foundation of psychoanalysis. Although Ireland firmly believed that "insanity in very young children is always accompanied or masked by idiocy,"[16] psychoanalysts, interested only in the former, saw no connection between the two. And by the late 1930s, American psychiatry was "largely living off the hypotheses coming from psychoanalysis," psychologist Alfred Baldwin reflected in a mid-century textbook, emphasizing the disciplinary shift in interest from genetics and heredity to "the effects of childhood experiences and environment upon the adult who emerges from these experiences."[17]

That was the nice way of putting it. But the language used by psychoanalysts was far less neutral; they explicitly (and often aggressively) blamed parents, especially mothers, for their kids' problems. In 1941, Margarethe Ribble proposed that inadequate mothering caused "serious privation reactions . . . which appear to be the basis of emotional disorders in the older child and in the adult."[18] Seven years later, Beata Rank argued that her young patients uniformly "suffered gross emotional deprivation" at the hands of a "dangerous mother" who was "emotionally disturbed," "narcissistic," and "immature."[19] That was the same year Frieda Fromm-Reichmann famously introduced the "schizophrenogenic mother," who created profound psychopathology through her "severe early warp and rejection" of her children.[20]

It's hard to imagine that many mothers were insulated from this chorus of voices identifying them as the "supreme mediator[s] of child development and social stability."[21] Psychoanalysis was featured in popular magazines like *Scientific American*, *Atlantic Monthly*, and *Life*.[22] Guidebooks for new parents, like Mary and C. Andrews Aldrich's *Babies Are Human Beings*, which was published in 1938, and Dr. Benjamin Spock's *Common Sense Book of Baby and Child Care*, which appeared eight years later, were based on psychoanalytic principles.[23] And the system of child guidance clinics—the multidisciplinary practices that treated the problem behavior of "normal" kids—had shifted its theoretical approach by the mid-1930s from an eclectic framework to a psychoanalytical paradigm that manifested in practice as "a stinging critique of mothers."[24]

But psychoanalysts don't deserve all the blame for creating the anti-mother climate of this period. This attitude reverberated through other academic disciplines, such as sociology—Ernest Groves described motherhood as "pathological"—and behaviorism: John Watson dedicated his guidebook on raising well-adjusted children "to the first mother capable of bringing up a happy son or daughter, but then proceeded to question the likelihood of such an event."[25] These perspectives converged with social concerns in the post–World War II era about how to put the working woman genie back in the heteronormative family bottle to provoke what John Neill has called "a deep misogyny [that] surfaced in American culture."[26]

What's clear is that, in the 1940s, a host of critics were emboldened to articulate very public and well-received attacks on mothers. Most notorious is novelist Philip Wylie's 1942 nonfiction bestseller *Generation of Vipers*, which was chosen by the American Library Association as one of the most important books of the first half of the twentieth century. Wylie offers a scathing account of "the destroying mother" who is "a human calamity" analogous to Hitler:

> [Mom] is a middle-aged puffin with an eye like a hawk that has just seen a rabbit twitch far below. She is about twenty-five pounds overweight, with no sprint, but sharp heels and a hard backhand. . . . She smokes thirty cigarettes a day, chews gum, and consumes tons of bonbons and petits fours. . . . She could not pass the final examinations of a fifth grader. . . . Nosing is not a mere psychological ornament of her; it is a basic necessity. . . . Knowing nothing about medicine, art, science, religion, law, sanitation, civics, hygiene, psychology, morals, history, geography, poetry, literature, or any other topic except the all-consuming one of momism.[27]

Four years later, psychiatrist Edward Strecker would cite Wylie approvingly in his own diatribe against mothers and "the emotional satisfaction, almost repletion, [they] deriv[e] from keeping [their] children paddling about in a kind of psychological amniotic fluid rather than letting them swim away with the bold and decisive strokes of maturity from the emotional maternal womb." Strecker specifically blamed mothers for schizophrenia, alcoholism, and homosexuality, but more generally he was concerned about a pervasive immaturity that, in compromising their sons' ability to serve as soldiers and leaders, threatened "the basic survival of the nation."[28] If this sounds hyperbolic, it wasn't just Wylie and Strecker: historian Anne Harrington notes that, in this period, "The failure of the mothers to love their children in the right way came to be seen as the witting or unwitting pernicious force behind virtually every form of deviant citizenship within society."[29]

* * *

Kanner's seminal paper introducing autism to the world was published the year after *Generation of Vipers*, but he had recognized and responded to mother-blaming trends well before then. Near the beginning of his 1941 book, *In Defense of Mothers: How to Bring Up Children in Spite of the More Zealous Psychologists*, he takes aim at his prime target:

> There is no raid shelter from the verbal bombs that rain on the contemporary parents. At every turn they run against weird words and phrases which are apt to confuse and scare them to no end: Oedipus complex, inferiority complex, maternal

> rejection, sibling rivalry, conditioned reflex, schizoid personality, repression, regression, aggression, blah-blah, blah-blah, and more blah-blah.[30]

In case a reader or two may have been living under a rock and failed to recognize those terms, Kanner later spells it out:

> The myth of the G.G.U. [Great God Unconscious] and his subdivisions has spread like wildfire. His religion is called psychoanalysis. . . . His altars are couches on which the worshippers, in recumbent position, are made to contemplate their spiritual navels, one hour each day or every other day, for a period of several years. Some day, when the G.G.U. will have changed His residence from the textbooks of psychology to those of mythology, parents will no longer be bothered about His mysterious vagaries. But at present they cannot escape His priests and believers.[31]

Kanner's book, in its savage, and often hilarious, shredding of psychoanalysis—which he further dismisses as "an unproven, arbitrarily decreed 'psychology,' sublimely removed from life as it is lived, scornful of facts and real occurrences"[32]—is highly entertaining reading. But more than that, his reassurance carried a lot of weight. Kanner, as historian Chloe Silverman reports, "virtually invented the specialty of child psychiatry"—he wrote the emerging discipline's first textbook in 1935, and he led Johns Hopkins University's Behavior Clinic for Children, which "became a model of its kind."[33] It was there that Kanner treated the eleven children whose shared "basic desire for aloneness and sameness" struck him as "markedly and uniquely [different] from anything reported so far"[34]—although the name he chose for it was not. Swiss psychiatrist Eugen Bleuler had actually introduced the word "autism" in 1911 to describe the profound withdrawal and detachment from reality he saw in his schizophrenic patients, and the term was widely used in the field.[35] By incorporating Bleuler's symptom in his new diagnosis, Kanner was foregrounding the children's "*inability to relate themselves* in the ordinary way to people and situations" (emphasis in original) as "fundamental" to the disorder.[36]

The bulk of Kanner's 1943 paper is composed of case reports documenting his patients' idiosyncratic or missing language, bizarre behavior, and inappropriate affect. But he did conclude with some thoughts about the possible cause of this new syndrome. Although Kanner had previously noted that the parents of all the children were both "highly intelligent . . . [with] very few really warmhearted fathers and mothers," the man who had defended parents from psychoanalysis was quick to absolve them once again: "The children's aloneness from the beginning of life makes it difficult to attribute the whole picture exclusively to the type of the early parental relations with our patients. . . . We must, then, assume that these children have come into the world with innate inability to form the usual, biologically provided affective contact with people."[37]

But this theory would soon change. By 1949, Kanner was arguing that "most of the patients were exposed from the beginning to parental coldness, obsessiveness, and a mechanical type of attention to material needs only. . . . They were kept neatly in refrigerators which did not defrost. Their withdrawal seems to be an act of turning away from such a situation to seek comfort in solitude."[38] This represents a monumental shift in Kanner's thinking. Not only was autism caused by parents—rather than being a condition that children were born with, as he had first hypothesized—but those parents were so terrible, so heartless, that their kids freely chose a life of incomprehensible, dangerous, and disabling symptoms rather than engage with them. And this was not a passing theory. In 1954, Kanner turned to the parents to answer the question with which he titled a paper: "To What Extent Is Early Infantile Autism Determined by Constitutional Inadequacies?" Not too much, he concluded. Not only did his patients have few psychotic relatives, which one would expect if heredity were to blame, but Kanner emphasized again the "emotional refrigeration" the children experienced at the hands of frigid mothers who offered "mechanized service of the kind which is rendered by an overconscientious gasoline station attendant."[39] And he used the same language at a 1955 symposium he presented with Leon Eisenberg, where he described "the common lot of autistic children" as one of "emotional refrigeration."[40]

Scholars have struggled to characterize Kanner's attitude toward parents—especially because, as we will see, he would later emphatically reject what would become known as the "refrigerator mother" theory of autism. Chloe Silverman references "ambiguities in his early writings [which] make it easy to see how readers interpreted his characterizations of parents as explicit claims about pathology and causation."[41] Professor of communication Majia Holmer Nadesan similarly describes Kanner's etiological theories as plagued by "ambiguity and ambivalence."[42] But his meaning seems perfectly clear to me. More compelling is the explanation offered by John Donvan and Caren Zucker in their history of autism—that Kanner, essentially, was swayed by peer pressure: "Calling autism inborn went against the main tide of thinking about mental illness. In the view of psychiatry, mental illness was always caused by traumatic emotional experiences, and mothers were almost always held to have played a part in the problem."[43]

Kanner wasn't the only one to capitulate; few could resist the reigning psychoanalytic theories of the time. Even the most prominent biological psychiatrists ultimately adopted them—including Bellevue Hospital's Lauretta Bender, who is best known today for using electroconvulsive therapy (ECT) in the 1940s to treat hundreds of schizophrenic children, some as young as three. Her choice of a somatic treatment like ECT reflected her belief that childhood schizophrenia was, as Kanner initially proposed about autism, inborn. As late as 1955 she was still arguing that the disorder was caused by "maturational lag at the embryonic level. . . . It is determined before birth, and hereditary factors appear to be the most important."[44] Bender always considered both biology and environment as important contributors to psychiatric disorders, but one short year later her emphasis had completely flipped: "Modern psychology no longer believes that any symptomatology is the direct result of a defect. . . . We have come to understand that the outstanding cause for behavior disorders in any child is deprivation in human relationships in the infantile period."[45] In 1959, she would describe autism as "a defense mechanism" in which children "withdraw or protect themselves from . . . disorganization and anxiety."[46]

This was pretty much how everyone described autism at mid-century—when, disability researcher Mitzi Waltz writes, "Freudian or 'psychodynamic' psychology provided the most prominent narrative of autism."[47] Louise Despert, for example, described a case study of an autistic son whose mother was "compulsive, perfectionistic, narcissistic, immature, frigid, emotionally detached, frightened by body contact, lacking in sensuousness, and capable of functioning satisfactorily only on an intellectual level." Despert reported satisfactorily that the boy was placed in a foster home; subsequently she strongly recommended that the family hire a nurse for their younger daughter, because "tender, emotional gratification from the mother was unavailable."[48]

Professor of English Jordynn Jack suggests that Kanner was particularly influenced by the work of John Bowlby, cited along with fellow psychoanalysts Despert, Margaret Mahler, and Beata Rank in the published version of that 1955 symposium.[49] Bowlby studied maternal deprivation during World War II and was charged by the World Health Organization with writing an influential report on his conclusions. After visiting clinics in both Europe and the United States, Bowlby reported that children who had been separated from their parents for any reason, including wartime relocation, hospitalization, or foster care, were more likely to present as apathetic and immature. He described the realization that "a warm, intimate, and continuous relationship with [a baby's] mother" is "essential for mental health" as "among the most significant developments in psychiatry during the past quarter of a century."[50]

Bowlby's work was itself informed by the emerging field of ethology, which examined animal behavior from a biological perspective. Rejecting classic psychoanalytic theories that located the origin of the mother-infant relationship in the breast as a source of nourishment or of oral fixation more broadly, Bowlby adapted Nikolaas Tinbergen's 1951 theory of instinct in animals, arguing instead for an evolutionary basis to a bond that dramatically increased a baby's chance of survival. For proof of his new framework, dubbed the theory of Component Instinctual Responses, Bowlby drew on the findings of a different ethologist, the American primate researcher Harry Harlow.[51]

Harlow's now notorious studies heartbreakingly demonstrated that comfort, not nutrition, was the motivating force behind infants' attachment to their mothers—at least for newborn macaque monkeys, who would cling to cloth-covered figures even if their food was provided by wire surrogates. Harlow's findings were enthusiastically picked up by the popular press—including the *Washington Post*, the *New York Times*, and *Life*—and he was invited to present on multiple television networks. The next year, he released an award-winning film of his experiments, *The Nature and Development of Affection*, that would become a mainstay of psychology courses going forward.

Particularly striking, especially for those interested in Kanner's relatively new diagnosis, was the behavior of the young monkeys. Even the macaques who had been raised with the cloth surrogates were "unexpectedly dysfunctional animals." Bruno Bettelheim—director of the Sonia Shankman Orthogenic School, a residential program for emotionally disturbed children at the University of Chicago, and the most vocal proponent of the "refrigerator mother" theory of autism—visited Harlow's lab at the University of Wisconsin in 1958 and "was struck by the rocking and pacing and self-clasping of the monkeys who had been raised with cloth mom. Their restless turning and hand-wringing reminded him immediately of his own autistic patients." Furthermore, as Bettelheim name-dropped in his bestselling 1967 book *The Empty Fortress*, Harlow's unresponsive surrogates reminded him of his patients' own frigid and loveless parents.[52]

Harlow would blast Bettelheim's analogy in an unpublished review of *The Empty Fortress*, arguing instead that "many autistic children are autistic because of brain malfunction in some unspecified or perhaps unspecifiable area."[53] But the similarities between his macaques and autistic children would prove irresistible to the ethology community. By 1969, in the first of three volumes elucidating what would be known as Attachment Theory, Bowlby was blaming inattentive, unpredictable, and neglectful mothers for "some forms of autism."[54] A few years later, Nikolaas Tinbergen would put aside his work with seagulls and honey bees to propose, along with his wife Elisabeth, a theory of autism that faulted "something in the behavior of the parents, in particular the mothers,"[55] and claimed dramatic results from an intervention of their own design, which combined forced eye contact with a type of holding therapy.[56] Even Harlow eventually admitted, despite his earlier attack on Bettelheim, that "the behavioral similarities between the isolate monkeys and autistic infants are striking," noting that both not only exhibited "marked social withdrawal," but "self-aggressive behaviors including self-biting and self-mutilation" as well.[57]

Later, more biologically inclined researchers would point out the obvious, as Uta Frith did in a 1984 critique of the Tinbergens' book: "Everyone would surely agree that a particular pattern of behaviour can arise from different causes. . . . It seems doubtful whether a single explanation for all the varieties of developmental social disorder is a useful aim."[58] But before then, few pointed out the fallacy of what seemed like a completely logical presumption: if total maternal deprivation could cause autistic behaviors, then autism more broadly must always be caused by maternal deprivation.

So is it any surprise that, even as parents of intellectually disabled children challenged stereotypes and stigma in popular memoirs of the 1950s and 1960s, the parents of children with autism and the often interchangeable diagnosis of childhood schizophrenia remained completely silent? Beyond the judgment of their kids' physicians, which might at least be confined to the examination room, it doubtlessly felt like they couldn't open a magazine or turn on the television without encountering Harlow's miserable, love-starved macaque babies or Bettelheim's comparison of autistic children to traumatized concentration camp prisoners. And the message was always the same. As Bettelheim solemnly states in *The Empty Fortress*—which was excerpted or profiled in some of the most prominent national publications, including the *New York Times*, the *New Yorker*, the *New Republic*, and *Time*—"The precipitating factor in infantile autism is the parent's wish that his child should not exist."[59]

That's not to say that no one was writing about such children during this period—but it wasn't the allegedly guilty parents, it was the therapists who were charged with saving them. In 1960, *Harper's Magazine* ran a photo essay featuring a young boy with childhood schizophrenia and his psychologist, Mira Rothenberg, "who is helping to unlock Jonny's strange prison," according to the introduction to the article. The parents are nowhere to be seen, but Rothenberg and Jonny are featured in several dark close-ups, allowing readers to witness Rothenberg's struggle to break through to a child she describes as "encapsulated from life and sound in his own private world."[60]

But the most popular narrative by far was psychologist Virginia Axline's 1964 account of, from the Introduction by Leonard Carmichael, "the emergence of a strong, healthy personality in a previously deeply disturbed child."[61] Axline names neither autism nor childhood schizophrenia explicitly in *Dibs in Search of Self*. But her five-year-old patient exhibits many classic autistic symptoms, including lack of eye contact, rocking, nonresponsiveness, violent temper tantrums, echolalia (the tendency to repeat what is heard), and pronoun reversal. And her assessment of the cause of Dibs's pathology echoes psychoanalytic understandings of these disorders. To be fair, Axline blames both cold parents for "the attacks upon [his personality]," that she believed catalyzed his retreat into autism, but only his mother's confession is described in detail: " 'My behavior was compulsive and completely unreasonable . . . I couldn't admit that I rejected him.' "[62]

Dibs was a tremendous and enduring bestseller—over the next fifteen years, more than 1.5 million copies would be sold, James Fisher reports, "expos[ing] millions of Americans to autism for the first time."[63] And what, exactly, did they learn? Not only that autism was caused by bad mothers—which was likely, at this point, unsurprising to readers—but that, in the hands of a compassionate and skilled therapist like Axline, the disorder's profound and disturbing symptoms could be rather quickly alleviated. Axline connects emotionally with Dibs during her first session with him; cures his pronoun reversal by his second visit; and discharges him completely cured after about a year of therapy with a newly tested IQ of 168, "an exceptionally gifted child."[64]

Recent research suggests, according to Mitzi Waltz, that "Dibs was at best a composite and exaggerated character, at worst a fictitious one."[65] But his "miraculous transformation"[66] helps us understand at least part of the reason why the parents of autistic children mutely, as science writer Edward Dolnick argues, "sat back and absorbed the blows." Organic problems, they thought, were incurable. But if they had done something to their previously normal children to cause autism, then it made sense that something else could be done to change them back: "Biology meant a life sentence without the possibility of parole," Dolnick concludes. "Psychology meant hope."[67]

* * *

Then, in 1967, Clara Claiborne Park published *The Siege: A Family's Journey into the World of an Autistic Child*. Why was she, finally, brave enough to challenge the hegemonic, mother-blaming discourse that cast parents not as advocates for their kids or partners to their physicians, but as the agents directly responsible for their children's autism?

Multiple factors likely contributed to Park's decision. First of all, this hegemony had very recently begun to crack. In 1964, psychologist Bernard Rimland (and parent of an autistic child himself) released *Infantile Autism: The Syndrome and Its Implications for a Neural Theory of Behavior*, which emphatically rejected psychogenic theories of etiology and argued that the disorder was caused by a physiological impairment. As we will see in the next chapter, Rimland's work would prove enormously influential in changing medical and lay understandings of autism. And Park not only read Rimland "with wonder,"[68] as she reports in *The Siege*, but she liked his book so much that she wrote to him the next day, starting a correspondence and collaboration that would lead to the founding of the National Society for Autistic Children in 1966.[69] Park did not always agree with Rimland, but she clearly considered him an ally in her opposition to the "parental rejection" claims she cites from Bettelheim, Rank, and Erik Erikson.[70]

Park's privilege as a white, married, upper-middle-class academic should also not be discounted. As other scholars have noted, disability parent memoirs in general have been primarily written by those with "the resources that allowed them to access, assess, and criticize the systems with which they interacted."[71] Park graduated from Radcliffe before earning a master's degree in English from the University of Michigan. She taught at a Massachusetts community college, wrote articles for the local newspaper, and was part of a lively intellectual community at Williams College, where her husband David was a physics professor. Although she clearly identified as an "amateur" in the autism world, these credentials likely made Park less intimidated by the "professionals" she encountered as she and David searched for help for their daughter Jessy (given the pseudonym Elly in the book), and less likely to submit to accusations that made no sense to her. How could her allegedly cold parenting cause Jessy's autism when her three older children were completely neurotypical? It couldn't, Park argued: "We were not disposed to blame ourselves. . . . We knew we had been the same kind of parents to Elly as we had been to the others. . . . Elly had been warmed, cuddled, tickled, and loved."[72]

This refutation was precisely the point. Waltz reports that the book "was written in part as a deliberate response to Bettelheim's work."[73] Marga Vicedo agrees: "Simply put, *The Siege* was to a large extent an act of self-defense, and a defense of other parents." And parents were tremendously receptive: Park's memoir "made waves throughout America"[74] and was translated into Spanish, French, German, Japanese, and several other languages.[75] But as much as she challenged the experts who blamed her for her daughter's autism, it is critical to note that Park did so in psychoanalytic language and imagery that fixed the intact mind in public conceptions of autism going forward.

It's right there in the title, *The Siege*, which also provides the guiding metaphor throughout the book, from the dedication—"To those behind walls, and to all their besiegers"—to this reflection in the closing chapter: "Of all the things that Elly has given, the most precious is this faith, a faith experience has almost transformed into certain knowledge: that inside the strongest citadel he can construct, the human being awaits his besieger."[76] This last sentence is indistinguishable from those written by prominent psychoanalysts, right down to the architectural metaphors—such as Margaret Mahler, who described "primary autism" as a condition in which "there is a deanimated, frozen wall between the subject and the human object."[77]

Also lifted straight from the psychoanalytic playbook is the implication that children *choose* to retreat into autism. For Park, this is a defining feature of the disorder—in her first description of it, she describes the paradigmatic affected child as "locked in himself, secure and satisfied in his repetitive activities, he will not use [his intelligence], or even display it for testing."[78] And her chapter names—including "Willed Weakness," "Willed Blindness," "Willed Deafness," and "Willed Isolation"—could have been crafted by Louise Despert, who emphasized, with italics, autistic children's "*determination not to communicate*"[79] or Axline's evocation of the "wall [Dibs] has built so sturdily around himself."[80]

To be clear, I am not suggesting that Park was a secret fan of psychoanalysis. In an interview decades later, she characterized psychoanalysts as "a bunch of failed poets," and that skcpticism is well evident in *The Siege*.[81] What I am arguing is that Park picked elements of reigning theories about autism that made sense to her and discarded the rest. Her quest to "attack, invade" Jessy's "solitary citadel" was largely self-directed initially, as Park experimented with strategies to teach her daughter to drink from a cup, complete a puzzle, or draw simple pictures. A visit from friends—a doctor and his wife—with an intellectually disabled son made her abandon her instinctively gentle approach and embrace "a certain kind of benevolent aggressiveness [that] was unexpectedly effective with Elly." A series of babysitters Park engaged when she went back to teaching utilized what she called "play therapy." And when a psychiatric consultation was recommended for their daughter, then age three and a half, Park scheduled one at a renowned children's hospital that she refers to as "the Institute," because she was determined to exhaust every option: "if we did not try psychiatry we would never be able to feel we had done all we could for Elly."[82] The Parks were directed to take Jessy for psychotherapy and were offered little else in the way of recommendations or prognoses by the Institute, but their experience with Anna Freud's Hampstead Clinic in England, where they lived for a year during David Park's sabbatical, was much more productive—especially when the assigned therapist stopped trying to treat Park and shifted her attention to Jessy, ultimately offering practical help like developing nonverbal forms of communication, resolving emergent toileting issues, and enrolling her in a nursery school.

This eclectic strategy would be overwhelmingly embraced in future parent memoirs. Autism lends itself particularly well to this approach because, as noted earlier, it was, and remains, such an unstable and uncertain diagnostic category that it's difficult to categorically rule anything out. As Park observed more than fifty years ago, perhaps her experience would have been different "if the professionals had access to a sure body of knowledge about psychotic or defective children, which they could have imparted to us. But they did not, nor did they pretend to." In practical terms, this meant that "conclusions drawn from [other children's] problems or solutions were of doubtful applicability to this particular child."[83]

The story of "this particular child" ends happily, with Park's declaration, "As a siege, it has been successful, for we have reached Elly."[84] What is less obvious is what exactly it means to stage a successful siege. More recent scholarship has wrestled with Park's use of this imagery and its connection to the cure narratives so prevalent in autism parent memoirs as a genre. Marga Vicedo argues that "Clara's metaphor of the siege did not refer to the effort to save a 'normal' withdrawn child," because "Jessy is not 'recovered' or 'saved' or 'cured.'"[85] Similarly, Jordynn Jack notes that "Park's narrative does not completely conform to the structure of the heroic quest . . . she does not claim recovery or a cure."[86] And it's true that Jessy hasn't lost her diagnosis by the final chapters, nor has she become indistinguishable from typical peers. She can't chatter easily with other children or interact with them appropriately. In fact, Park clearly states, "The expectation of cure is a luxury we have learned to do without."[87]

Neither, however, has the hope been completely abandoned. Not only has Jessy already made tremendous progress—from the almost-two-year-old at the beginning of *The Siege* who couldn't walk, talk, pretend, or engage with anyone, to an eight-year-old who can draw maps, pretend her dolls are going to the supermarket, and stroke her mother while joking about her being "furry"[88]—but Park has resolved a question that plagued her throughout the narrative: Is Jessy intellectually disabled? Early in the book, she admitted that her daughter seemed "retarded in what she did" and rhetorically asked, "Why should we imagine that her retardation was 'different'?"[89]

Why? Because Jessy's diagnosis of autism technically precluded intellectual disability, at least in the period covered by *The Siege*. Remember that Kanner had ascribed "good cognitive potentialities" to all his young patients in his paper introducing autism to the world—even though, as he noted about one subject, "his incoherent speech, inability to conform, and reaction with temper outbursts to any interference created the impression of feeblemindedness," while another "was thought to be seriously retarded in intellectual development" because he was completely nonverbal and spent hours shredding cardboard boxes. Although the IQ of almost half the children couldn't actually be tested because they would not or could not cooperate with the examiners, Kanner's initial conviction that, as a colleague had reported about one seven-year-old girl, "'Without a doubt . . . her intelligence is superior to this,'"[90] led him to bake the intact mind right into his new syndrome.

And, in fact, by the end of *The Siege*, Park's worry has been assuaged: "[Jessy] is not feeble-minded; her mind, for those aspects of the world she can make sense of, is sharp and retentive."[91] This doesn't mean she is completely "normal." She still can't ride a bike, tie her shoes, or follow a complicated story. But the future is hopeful. In the penultimate chapter, Park recounts a story that Jessy's psychiatrist told her about a boy "who seemed much like [Jessy] and who ended up at Harvard." Picking up on the theme she had raised earlier about the uncertainty of autism, Park muses, "Neither he, nor we, nor anyone else knows what will become of her. The most we can say is that at one time the prognosis was nearly hopeless, and that now there is no prognosis at all."[92]

But most fundamentally, Vicedo's alternative interpretation of the "siege" of Jessy's "walled personality"[93] as "the family's work teaching Jessy the skills necessary for her to function in a world she found chaotic"[94] ignores both the larger psychoanalytic context of Park's metaphors as well as her own rhetorical strategy. It wasn't just Mahler and Axline who, as cited earlier, used the same metaphor of a wall to describe the pathology of autism and childhood schizophrenia—this imagery was pervasive in the psychoanalytic theories of autism that were so prevalent while Park was writing. Beata Rank described "thick walls built out of hatred and fear"[95]; Frances Tustin imagined autistic children as "encapsulated" by autistic "barriers."[96] And everyone knew what was on the other side: Edward Dolnick summarizes, "The common feature of all such theories was the belief that, behind their glass wall, autistic children were normal."[97]

If there was any doubt—despite the many, many references to walls and breaches and citadels and fortifications—about what exactly was at stake, Park also offers a different analogy, one she had to know would resonate with her readers: even those who knew nothing about autism, schizophrenia, or psychoanalysis would recognize her reference to "the waiting child inside the lonely little wild animal that was Helen Keller."[98] And she doesn't just raise this comparison once—Park mentions her study of the biography of Annie Sullivan four separate times. Given this context, it's difficult to accept any other interpretation of what a successful siege would look like for Park short of the recovery of her daughter's intact mind.

* * *

The intact mind was one of Park's most impactful legacies and can be found in most of the parent memoirs about severely autistic children that followed—even those in which little progress is made, and the children remain at the end significantly impaired. In 1971, Joan Martin Hundley—an Australian whose memoir *The Small Outsider* was published in the United States—recounts a presentation her husband gave to a "kindergarten mothers' club," in which he describes life with an autistic child as " 'the feeling that the child is cut off by a "glass wall," that his mind is beyond our reach.' "[99] And while the book ends with a tender scene between Hundley and her son David, now six, during which she reflects, "I think little David would like to join the world of people. If only he can find the way," he remains nonverbal and prone to flushing his mother's manuscript pages down the toilet and eloping from his house "wearing his sister's nightie or naked . . . [and] wearing rubber gloves on his feet."[100]

Much more well-known is Josh Greenfeld's 1972 memoir, *A Child Called Noah*, the first of what would become a trilogy about his severely autistic son. Greenfeld's tone is more blunt, even bitter at times. Despite several intensive and expensive interventions—including moving across the country for several months so four-year-old Noah could be treated at the University of California, Los Angeles (UCLA), by O. Ivar Lovaas, who famously pioneered the use of behaviorism in autistic children—he makes minimal gains. Although he can say a word or two, and is partially toilet-trained, Noah still requires so much energy, instruction, and supervision that Greenfeld and his wife, both writers, despair of ever having enough time to pursue their creative endeavors: "I must confess something," he writes: "Sometimes I hope Noah gets sick and dies painlessly."[101]

Not a very Park-like declaration. And Greenfeld's conclusion that all autistic children are "brain damaged," and his resignation that "there will never be one big gestalt of a miracle—one's secret dream, one's treasured notion—a dramatic breakthrough with an organ chord string," would seem to make him an unlikely apostle of the intact mind. Yet this short volume, not even 200 pages long, references it multiple times. Greenfeld muses about his son, for example, "There is an opaque barrier, a filter or a jell, that he places between himself and the world," a state that changes little, as he notes later: "Noah is still very much enclosed in a world of his own whose latch he makes not even the slightest attempt to jiggle."[102]

There are other similarities as well between these two early memoirs. Like Park, the initial lack of medical consensus around his son's problems leaves Greenfeld and his wife Foumi in a constant state of uncertainty: "We'd been told he was mentally retarded; emotionally disturbed; autistic; schizophrenic;

possibly brain-damaged; or that he was suffering from a Chinese-box combination of these conditions." Even after Noah received his diagnosis, there was no agreement about the proper course of treatment. Psychotherapy was recommended for Greenfeld and Foumi on multiple occasions; they also pursued high-dose vitamin therapy for Noah, as well as the intensive behavioral intervention already described. With no clear prognosis or intervention, it seems, hope for the intact mind is impossible to suppress—even for a skeptic like Greenfeld, who dutifully reports the regressions that often followed Noah's slow and small accomplishments. Interestingly, Greenfeld also evokes the same paradigmatic emblem as Park, comparing his son to Helen Keller in one passage, and his family to "miracle workers" in another.[103] The resonance of Keller's story for parents of severely autistic children seems surprising at first, since she is overwhelmingly associated in the public mind with sensory deficits that are not typically found in this population. But for these parents, Keller's blindness and deafness were secondary to her sudden transformation, the discovery of the intact mind in someone whose behaviors had marked her as severely cognitively impaired.

For Noah, the intact mind would never be recovered. In fact, this failure would lead Greenfeld to reject his son's diagnosis in his 1978 sequel, *A Place for Noah*. "By far the cruelest effect of the glamorous term *autism* is the specious hope it promises for a miracle cure," he writes. "I no longer consider—or call—my son Noah autistic. . . . [He] is brain damaged. . . . Encircling him with an Orwellian word such as autism—one that cosmeticizes rather than communicates—is no help."[104] But two other memoirs from this period describe a very different outcome. *For the Love of Ann*, published in 1973, and *Son-Rise*, which appeared three years later, are the first autism parent memoirs to claim recovery based on particular interventions.

For the Love of Ann is not technically a memoir, because it was written by Scottish journalist James Copeland. But because Copeland based his account on the diary of Ann's father, Jack Hodges (who is credited as a second author), as well as interviews with the family, it seems likely the book was received similarly to the autism parent memoirs of the period by readers who may have learned about it from the *Reader's Digest* Book Section, where it was featured.

As a toddler, Ann was profoundly impaired. She was completely nonverbal and spent hours rocking, always in one particular chair, "then she would bang her head against the wall, and scream if anyone tried to stop her. She pulled her hair out in handfuls and stuffed it in her mouth." She didn't respond to her name, did not want to be held by her parents, and refused to play with other children, including her two brothers, who considered her a "snarling, spitting animal."[105]

As disturbing as those behaviors were, the recovery of Ann's intact mind is foreshadowed very early—on the first page of the book, for those who peeked inside the cover to read the excerpt chosen to entice bookstore browsers: "Jack sat in his deck-chair and pondered on the problem for hours. . . . There must be a key somewhere. If they could find it, then they could unlock the door to that troubled mind."[106]

It's obvious why *For the Love of Ann* did not have the staying power of *The Siege*. Even though Ann ends up "beat[ing] autism," the "key" Jack finds would shock contemporary readers: "It had been accidental violence that had ended Ann's fear of sand and water. Now if they were to use DELIBERATE violence—by smacking her every time she did something they did not want her to do—would it not have the same effect?" Ann's mother Ivy reluctantly agrees to this strategy when Jack pleads, "Surely [she] would not deny him the chance of unlocking the door?"[107]

Over the course of the book, Ann is hit when she refuses to use a spoon, when she rocks, when she intentionally breaks eggs at the grocery store, and when she inappropriately touches strangers on the bus. And it works. Marveling at the changes in his daughter after just a month of contingent punishment, later paired with positive reinforcement for good behavior, Jack "was now sure that there was a considerable amount of intelligence in that little being waiting to be released."[108]

As Ann's behaviors decrease, the family works on teaching her to talk, to count, and to read, until she is able to join a local special education class. By the age of eighteen, "she had progressed from a hopeless, speechless, screaming walking vegetable to an attractive teenager who could read, write and spell as well as many normal children of her age. She had a thirst for knowledge that could not be quenched." Her conversation, Copeland assures us, is completely typical, reflecting her desire to become a wife and mother. The story ends with Ann on a vacation to Spain, where she "joined in the fiestas and went to nightclubs, dancing until dawn."[109]

Son-Rise, by Barry Kaufman, depicts a similar, but much condensed, trajectory. At the beginning of the book, Kaufman's son Raun seems very similar to Jessy Park, Noah Greenfeld, or Ann Hodges. When he was eighteen months old, he had no language and was so disengaged from his family that doctors suspected he might be deaf. After receiving little medical help and rejecting therapeutic programs based on psychoanalysis and behaviorism, Kaufman and his wife Suzi decide to create their own therapeutic model based on the Option Method, "which was born out of the Option Attitude: 'To love is to be happy with.' " This entrepreneurial approach was necessary, Kaufman argued, because experts clearly didn't have the answers: "Two generations of research and energy had produced elaborate systems of judgments and predictions," he states. "And yet, for all this effort, little had transpired that was meaningful for this small boy and others like him."[110]

The Kaufmans' home-grown program had three stages. First, the family spent hours joining Raun in activities that today would be called "self-stimulatory," such as spinning and rocking, to show him that "he was accepted and approved of." Next came a "motivational" phase that, similar to Park's approach with Jessy, was designed to encourage Raun to choose "our world" over his autistic solitude. The final step borrowed from principles of behaviorism and broke down skills and tasks (like completing puzzles and building block towers) into component parts for easier instruction.[111] In order to eliminate distractions, Kaufman and Suzi conducted what would turn into thousands of hours of therapy in their bathroom.

That was the methodology. But the goal was, as always, to recover the intact mind—the existence of which Kaufman never questions. He describes his toddler son as "encapsulated," and his fear that Raun would be "lost behind an impenetrable barrier . . . wandering alone in the recesses of his head and searching for a passageway that would never be there." When Raun seems to become more socially engaged, Kaufman celebrates his "breaking through the walls," and when he seems withdrawn, his father worries that "we had lost him behind that invisible and impenetrable wall." At his most explicit, Kaufman connects the dots, explaining that all the activities "were going have more impact beyond just motivating and socializing" because they would create "an opening on the surface . . . [for] the depths of [Raun's] mind."[112]

Raun is only two years old when *Son-Rise* ends, but the battle has already been won: Kaufman reports that, after seven months of intensive therapy, his son "had found the new pathways [and] opened new channels" to successfully move "through the barrier of his own encapsulation." The final scene is one that will be repeated, with different players, in many future autism parent memoirs: the re-evaluation of the child by medical experts who had once found him profoundly impaired. Four months earlier, Kaufman reports, Raun's language and socialization skills placed him at the level of an eight-month-old. Now, at the age of two, "in over half the tests, Raun functioned at the thirty-to-thirty-six-month level. . . . The doctors were dramatically impressed and surprised."[113]

The following years would be quiet ones for autism parent memoirs. Few new examples would appear until the 1990s, when a "surge" of autism parent memoirs would begin that is still ongoing.[114] By that time, medical thinking about the disorder had changed dramatically. Autism was no longer considered a form of psychosis but a developmental disorder, and biological theories of causation had consolidated a decade earlier among the most prominent researchers and clinicians, who all agreed that autism was both physiologically based and incurable. British psychiatrist Michael Rutter had challenged the intact mind narrative as early as 1965: "It has sometimes been thought that all autistic children are 'really' of normal intelligence, and that intellectual brilliance always exists beneath the autistic surface of failures to speak, learn and form relationships. Regrettably, this is not the case."[115]

Not that you would know it by reading these second-generation memoirs. Even as they embraced biological theories and universally looked back on Bruno Bettelheim and the "refrigerator mother" as the epitome of the Autism Dark Ages, parent-authors never let go of the intact mind. Surgically severed from the psychoanalytic ideas that shaped it, this concept proved extraordinarily malleable, surfacing in accounts that celebrated everything from alternative therapies to cutting-edge genetic research. No matter what interventions were pursued, or whether or not they worked, if there is one thread that connects autism parent memoirs from *The Siege* to the present, it's that no outcome is more desired, no fight is harder fought, no loss is more keenly mourned, than that of the intact mind.

3

Is There a "Key"?

Biomedical Discourse and Second-Generation Autism Memoirs, 1980s–Present

It's unclear why hardly any autism parent memoirs were published in the 1980s. English professor Julie Rak has identified a general "memoir boom" in the years surrounding the new millennium,[1] but there were other factors specific to autism that doubtlessly contributed to the flood of autism parent memoirs starting in the early 1990s. Sociologists Claire Laurier Decoteau and Meghan Daniel point to the growth of advocacy organizations, national conferences, and CDC surveillance in this decade as a disciplinary cornerstone, the moment when "autism began to emerge as the main concern of a nascent field."[2]

How much the public was attending to these events is debatable. But what is indisputable is the impact that one movie had on American awareness and interest in autism: *Rain Man*, which was released in 1988 and won four Academy Awards, including Best Picture and Best Actor for Dustin Hoffman, who played autistic savant Raymond Babbitt. Numerous scholars have pointed to the film as a key moment in autism discourse, including Stuart Murray, who calls *Rain Man* "the foundational text for all the various contemporary representations of autism, the breakthrough story that gave the condition a public profile when before it was, to a large degree, confined to medical and educational specialists, and the families of those individuals who had autism."[3]

Rain Man's immense popularity—it was the top-grossing movie of the year—doubtlessly contributed to the rush of autism parent memoirs that would shortly begin. But perhaps even more important were the profound changes in medical thinking about the disorder. Although *The Empty Fortress* received much attention in the mainstream media, from a medical perspective it represented the last gasp of psychoanalytic theories of autism causation. Even before its publication, Bernard Rimland's *Infantile Autism* had emphatically rejected psychogenic explanations that blamed parents for their children's often profound deficits in language, behavior, and social engagement.

Although Rimland's specific hypothesis of "the reticular system [of the brain] as a site for the conceptual impairment"[4] was never embraced by researchers and clinicians, a broader consensus quickly developed in the medical community that autism was both biological and intractable. In 1965, Michael Rutter argued that "some form of damage or injury to the brain is an important factor in the development of child psychosis or autism. . . . The condition is not to be blamed on the way that the parents have brought up the child."[5] Five years later, his compatriot Lorna Wing laid out the reasons why "refrigerator mother" theories of autism were not compelling:

> Firstly, systematic studies of parents have not shown anything unusual in their personalities apart from the problems common to parents of handicapped children in general. . . . Secondly, most of these parents have other children who are quite normal. . . . Thirdly, none of the excellent studies of old-fashioned institutions, where babies really were deprived of all maternal care, has shown that they caused early childhood autism.[6]

Empirical reports of specific physiological abnormalities in autistic children also began to accumulate in the 1960s, such as elevated serotonin levels,[7] irregular electroencephalogram (EEG) patterns,[8] and the high prevalence of epilepsy in this population, affecting approximately 17% of autistic adolescents.[9]

By 1971, American psychologist Eric Schopler was publishing a scathing indictment of Bettelheim and his colleagues in the *Journal of Contemporary Psychotherapy*. In the bluntly titled "Parents of Psychotic Children as Scapegoats," Schopler hypothesized that psychoanalytically oriented clinicians blamed parents to alleviate their own "feelings of inferiority" in the face of a puzzling disorder with outcomes that were, at best, "uneven"—circumstances under which "the clinician's role as an authoritative expert is seriously threatened."[10]

Even Kanner, who had coined the devastating "refrigerator mother" epithet and waffled about the causes of autism for more than a quarter of a century, had finally made up his mind. In 1969, at the inaugural meeting of the National Society for Autistic Children, Kanner stepped to the podium and declared to the audience, in a statement that reverberated through the autism community, "Herewith I acquit you people as parents."[11]

This position was not entirely unanimous. As late as 1992, British psychotherapist Frances Tustin was defending her psychoanalytically infused belief that "the traumatic stress which had provoked the autistic reactions had been experiences of unbearably sudden and painful awareness of bodily separateness from a mother with whose body they had previously felt fused and equated." In other words, Tustin proposed, autism was provoked by "unmitigated terror" and should be considered similar to post-traumatic stress disorder.[12]

But if parents read Tustin, they certainly didn't write about it. Instead, Bruno Bettelheim would continue to play the role of supervillain in autism parent memoirs. Annabel Stehli's account of her discovery of Bettelheim's theories—which she describes as "the most profoundly unsettling news I'd ever had"—takes up several pages of her 1991 book *The Sound of a Miracle*. "Bettelheim was accusing me of a vast hidden agenda," she reports, "a kind of passive infanticide."[13] The next year, Judy Barron remembered the cultural climate when her own son was newly diagnosed, in which the director of the Orthogenic School was so famous everyone knew his name: " 'You've read Bettelheim,' a friend tells Barron after she asks for a referral to a psychologist. " 'You know what the current thinking is: *The mother did it!*' "[14] And in *News from the Border*, published in 1993, Jane Taylor McDonnell recalls her emotional reaction to *The Empty Fortress*, which was one of the only titles relating to autism at her local library: "I was shaking. Was I worse than an SS guard? Had I destroyed my child in the most callous and brutal way imaginable?"[15]

These parents were largely recounting how it felt to read Bettelheim at the height of his influence, in the 1960s and 1970s. But by the end of the century, when they wrote their memoirs, his name evoked anger and contempt, not guilt. Not only had psychoanalysis been largely rejected by the psychiatric profession, but shocking revelations followed Bettelheim's 1990 suicide: that he held a PhD in art history, not psychology, and his primary employment before his immigration to the United States had involved managing his family's lumber business. Even worse than fabricating his psychoanalytic credentials, Bettelheim had abused his young patients and misrepresented their outcomes.[16] The "respected authority"[17] that Annabel Stehli couldn't bring herself to doubt, the name that Patricia Stacey's professors "evoke[d] . . . with reverence,"[18] the expert whose "wisdom and compassion" was celebrated in the *New York Times*[19]—was a fraud.

But Bettelheim's exposure did not mitigate his influence. His betrayal was so profound that it catalyzed a distrust of the medical establishment that persists among many autism parents to this day—even though, as noted earlier, by the time second-generation memoirists were writing, clinicians and researchers had firmly rejected psychogenic models of autism etiology in favor of biological theories. Instead of blaming parents, some prominent practitioners even engaged them as allies. Bernard Rimland both solicited their feedback in a questionnaire included in *Infantile Autism* and joined with prominent parent advocates (including Clara Claiborne Park) to form the National Society for Autistic Children in 1965.[20] And when University of North Carolina researchers Eric Schopler and Robert Reichler developed what would become the first statewide autism intervention program, TEACCH (Treatment and Education of Autistic and Communication-related Handicapped Children) during this same period, they explicitly embraced parents as necessary and effective therapists for their children.[21]

This realignment should theoretically have left physicians and families on the same side. But the new medical model of autism etiology carried a decidedly unwelcome prognosis. As discussed in the previous chapter, many parents did not push back against psychogenic theories because they at least allowed for the possibility of recovery. Hypotheses of abnormal brain development, however, were much more pessimistic. Michael Rutter's unequivocal rejection of the intact mind was echoed in a British Medical Association pamphlet published in 1970 by Lorna Wing: "Most parents of these children have the feeling that their child is potentially normal and intelligent, if only they could find the key to the mystery of his strange behavior . . . [but] most [autistic children] have learning problems that make them generally retarded."[22] Later that decade, American psychiatrist Marian DeMyer similarly criticized the pervasive assumption that "all autistic children . . . [have] the capacity for accelerating in intellectual progress and finally becoming normal or nearly so if the right treatment key can be found" because most cases end "tragically in an adult life of partial or total dependence."[23] And this conviction was not restricted to researchers and other academics. In his memoir *Without Reason*, Charles Hart recounts the speech that accompanied his son Ted's autism diagnosis in 1978. "Let me give you a warning," the doctor told Hart and his wife Sara. "There is no 'key' to unlock your child from his disability. There is no normal little human being hiding behind some mask of autism."[24]

Smarting from decades of parent blaming, and reeling from the grim foreclosure of their children's futures, parent-authors from the end of the twentieth century to the present decisively pushed back, privileging their own expertise over that of their children's practitioners. Judy Barron remembers the resolution she and her husband made following a disappointing visit to a nutritionist: "We were going to depend on ourselves from now on. We'd fight for Sean our way, and if we were wrong, the mistakes would be ours."[25] Cheri Florance despairs, in her 2004 memoir, at the experts who saw in her son Whitney "a severely retarded child with multiple handicaps in his physical abilities and his communication and his intelligence" while "the mother in me saw a future engineer en route to MIT."[26] Even in 2020, thirty years after Bettelheim's death, Marcia Hinds was using derisive quotation marks to indicate her opinion of the "experts" that predicted her son Ryan would "probably end up in an institution. . . . Without discussion, my husband and I decided we would not accept what this expert said."[27]

Occasionally parents offered their credentials as proof that their decision to dismiss their doctors' recommendations wasn't completely ignorant or irrational. In the introduction to her 2015 memoir about her son Ben, Susan Levin announces, "I am a Harvard College graduate."[28] And Cheri Florance repeatedly references her PhD in speech and language pathology, particularly to support her conclusion that her son Whitney never really had autism, as he was diagnosed, but suffered instead from a previously unrecognized sensory disorder that she proposes to call "the Florance Maverick Syndrome."[29]

But much more common is the assertion that parental expertise trumps medical orthodoxy, even in the absence of fancy diplomas. In her 2007 book *Louder than Words*, actress and former Playboy bunny Jenny McCarthy proudly proclaims her degree from "the University of Google."[30] Bill Davis never even went to college. Unlike most authors of autism parent memoirs—or memoirs in general—the author of 2001's *Breaking Autism's Barriers* does not have a wealthy or educated background; he is a high school graduate who works as a bartender. But he becomes such a prominent advocate that he is routinely contacted by other parents for advice and is invited to educate local law enforcement about autism. He knows his tattoos and his wife Jae's piercings undermine conventional assumptions about what authorities are supposed to look like, but he has no patience for "so-called experts" who "are too full of theory"—and, he writes, he is not alone. At one autism conference, Davis and his wife sat on a panel with "PhDs and an audience of educators. . . . [But] every question [following the panel] was directed to Jae and me." Ultimately, Davis is less concerned with readers making the exact same decisions that he and Jae did regarding their son Chris's care than he is with empowering them to "decide for yourself which therapy and education is good for [your child] rather than what other people offer or tell you, and then go get it."[31]

Of course, skepticism toward the medical profession is hardly unique to autism parents. Paul Starr, in his classic history of medicine in the United States, traces this discontent to the 1970s, and credits the women's movement in particular with rebelling against "paternalistic doctors who refused to share information or take [women's] intelligence seriously" and, more fundamentally, "object[ing] that much of what passed for scientific knowledge was sexist prejudice."[32] This challenge to medical authority was echoed by contemporaries like anti-psychiatry advocate Thomas Szasz, who claimed there was no such thing as mental illness; epidemiologist Thomas McKeown, who credited population growth in the nineteenth century to improvements in nutrition, sanitation, and reproductive control rather than medical innovation; and philosopher Ivan Illich, who believed that modern medicine just made people sicker. Political scientist Tom Nichols argues for an even broader, society-wide "death of expertise" originating in this period, and posits that the particularly American conviction that all opinions are equally valid has only intensified over the subsequent decades.[33] Still, autism as a disorder seems especially conducive to this mindset—due not only to the reasons discussed above, but to other factors that differentiated autism parent memoirs from accounts of raising children with other types of intellectual and developmental disabilities.

First, unlike kids with Down syndrome or cerebral palsy, autistic children typically carry no physical markers of their disability. And not only are they free from such stigmata, but their exceptional beauty is a common theme in these memoirs. Marcia Hinds reports that "Ryan was one of the best-looking boys in his class."[34] Annabel Stehli explains that this is not unusual: "As is typical of autistic children, [her daughter Georgie] was exceptionally beautiful, with her blue eyes offset by dark lashes, and her hair a mass of silky curls."[35] Charlotte Moore elaborates, "[Autistic children] are outstandingly good-looking—much better-looking than one would expect from observing their parents. . . . Sam is a handsome, well-knit boy, with glossy dark hair, an elegant neck, and a rather haughty expression, almost like an Indian brave. . . . George is a high-cheekboned beauty, with luminous eyes, like a super-model on drugs."[36]

Jane Taylor McDonnell reflects, "It surprised me a little that this physical beauty should mean so much to me."[37] But it shouldn't have. Physiognomics—as classicist Elizabeth Evans defines it, "the art of interpreting character from the physique"—dates back to the ancient world. Hippocrates, Galen, Aristotle, and Homer, among many others, thought that intelligence, bravery, and integrity could be discerned from the face and body, as could undesirable attributes such as insanity.[38] Eighteenth-century Europeans firmly believed that "idiocy was something you could see marked on the face and body of the person who carried it"—but anyone in need of assistance interpreting the particular signs could always consult one of the fifty-five editions of Johann Kaspar Lavater's *Essays on Physiognomy* that were published between 1789 and 1810.[39] For disability scholars David Mitchell and Sharon Snyder, the disabled "have always been subject to varieties of this interpretive practice."[40]

In other words, physical beauty meant so much because it was closely tied in the cultural imagination to the intact mind. Moore—one of the few parent-authors whose children don't recover, whose sons are "autistic through and through"—sagely notes that "whether we admit it or not, we are hugely affected by physical appearances. Despite plenty of evidence to the contrary, we associate good looks with intelligence. . . . Autistic beauty augments the fairy-tale feeling that the child is in suspended animation, enclosed just out of reach in glass or ice."[41] But most parents were not so self-aware, assuring themselves, as Jack Hodges did decades earlier in the diaries that would become *For the Love of Ann*, "A child as beautiful as Ann could NOT be a mental defective. It didn't add up. It didn't make sense. Mental defectives had that certain look about them."[42]

Furthermore, autistic children don't always *act* cognitively impaired. Many exhibit splinter skills—narrow areas of typical or even exceptional ability—that can result in very uneven developmental profiles. Charles Hart reports that his son Ted's "IQ ranged from a low of 20 in speech and social skills up to 120 in academic ability."[43] My own son Jonah, as mentioned earlier, was hyperlexic, able to read and write at a very young age. So was Robert Hughes's son Walker, whose ability, at the age of four, to spell words like "helicopter" that he was unable to say led Hughes and his wife Ellen to refer to him as their "eccentric genius."[44] Bill Davis describes his shock when his two-year-old son Chris "set up A through Z with his plastic letters," which impressed Davis and his wife Jae as "amazingly smart" even as they struggled to stop Chris from screaming, flapping his hands, spinning objects, and "eating the wood on the table."[45]

A small percentage of autistics do demonstrate such incredible talents in domains like music or math that they are classified as savants—like Raymond Babbit, *Rain Man*'s protagonist, who displays astonishing abilities counting cards at a blackjack table and calculating the exact number of toothpicks in a jumble on the floor, although he is ultimately unable to thrive outside his structured and supported institutional environment. But savantism is extraordinarily rare, affecting no more than 1% of autistic individuals.[46] Even so, Stuart Murray argues, following the success of *Rain Man*, "the figure of the autistic savant presented as the normative mode of autistic subjectivity."[47] The public, in short, assumed that all autistics were also savants.

A third factor that emboldened parents was that autism was no more stable a diagnosis than it was in the mid-twentieth century. If anything, it was less. While Kanner had insisted on a narrow set of diagnostic criteria—even while lamenting that these weren't stringently applied—in 1981 Lorna Wing introduced the world to the work of Austrian psychiatrist Hans Asperger and the idea of the autism *spectrum*.[48] Asperger had actually published his paper identifying what he thought was a new syndrome, autistic psychopathy, in 1944—just one year after Kanner proposed his shockingly similar diagnosis of autistic disturbances of affective contact—but the advent of World War II prevented the translation and dissemination of his work. Although Asperger's subjects, unlike some of Kanner's, were fully verbal, the children shared other important symptoms: impaired social interaction, inappropriate use of language, and rigid and repetitive behaviors. Both researchers also observed the preponderance of affected boys as compared to girls.

In 2015, journalist Steve Silberman challenged this long-assumed coincidence. In his bestselling autism history *NeuroTribes*, Silberman argued that Kanner stole the idea of autism from Asperger—a theft allegedly facilitated by physician Georg Frankl, a former colleague of Asperger's who had fled the Nazis and later worked with Kanner at Johns Hopkins.[49] Historian Edith Sheffer repudiated this theory three years later, concluding that "the idea of autism was not considered to be Asperger's." Instead, she identifies Frankl and his wife, psychologist Anni Weiss, as the first true autism experts, having "both described the typology in more well-known scholarly publications than had Asperger—in 1934, 1935, and 1937."[50] And Kanner didn't steal from them either. As Sheffer notes, he cited them in his own articles.

For our purposes, all that matters from this story is that, by including Asperger's higher-functioning patients in her proposed spectrum, Wing effectively expanded the boundaries of the disorder, from "profound mental retardation"—no longer, as Kanner considered it, mutually exclusive—right up to "mildly eccentric variations of typical development."[51] This new framework—emphasizing what Wing called the "triad of impairments," namely, problems with social reciprocity, communication, and rigidity[52]—dramatically increased the number of kids who were diagnosed. Although researchers had previously estimated autism prevalence at "2–5 in 10,000," by 1994 Wing had suggested that as many as 1% of all children might be affected.[53] Six years later, she would compare her introduction of Asperger's syndrome to the opening of Pandora's Box and admit that "controversy over definitions of subgroups and prevalence of autistic spectrum disorders has increased."[54]

These constantly shifting boundaries and diagnostic criteria only increased the uncertainty articulated by Clara Claiborne Park and Josh Greenfeld in the 1960s and early 1970s. Marcia Hinds, describing the landscape circa 1993, noted that "not many of the 'experts' agreed about anything. There were many conflicting theories about autism."[55] Agreed Bill Davis, "There was not even a definitive test for autism, only a checklist of symptoms. . . . The specialists essentially admitted they didn't know much about autism."[56] Although medical researchers could celebrate significant findings—such as Susan Folstein and Michael Rutter's 1977 twin study establishing a genetic component in autism,[57] or the discoveries of abnormalities in autistic brains reported by multiple teams using new neuroimaging tools in the 1980s[58]—these advancements offered nothing in the way of practical help for parents. Noted Charles Hart in

1989, "Empirical research with large populations and careful evaluations had done nothing for [autistic children]. . . . [Parents] felt abandoned by the FDA and the AMA. [They] wanted solutions and [were] prepared to take risks."[59]

And they increasingly turned to other parents for those solutions, because—and this is the final and most important factor behind the alienation of so many autism parents from the medical establishment—the parents, if the growing catalog of memoirs could be believed, were right. Even as doctors repeatedly stressed that the often profound cognitive impairments exhibited by many autistic children were irremediable, parent-authors in book after book celebrated the recovery of the intact mind—often accompanied by detailed instructions on how they accomplished what their kids' own doctors predicted would never happen.

Occasionally, these narratives featured orthodox interventions. Both *Let Me Hear Your Voice*, by Catherine Maurice, and *Autism: From Tragedy to Triumph*, by Carol Johnson and Julia Crowder, describe the transformation of autistic children through the use of the behavior modification therapy developed by UCLA psychologist Ole Ivar Lovaas. In 2019, Applied Behavior Analysis (ABA)—the catchall phrase eventually attached to therapies such as Lovaas's based on the principles of operant conditioning—would become the first autism intervention covered by insurance in all 50 states, because it was one of the few supported by empirical evidence.[60] But the claims of ABA practitioners have moderated considerably since Lovaas's 1987 paper announcing the complete recovery of almost half the young autistic subjects in his experimental group, who all received forty hours or more of individualized behavior therapy a week.[61]

Maurice's children, Anne-Marie and Michel, and Crowder's son Drew fall into that category, and their mothers' memoirs (published within a year of one another in the early 1990s) follow the pattern set by Park and Greenfeld—Maurice actually cites Park's influence, recounting her experience reading *The Siege*: "As I read on that night, two concepts fairly burst into my consciousness: the notion of Anne-Marie as being 'walled in,' and the idea of assaulting those ramparts."[62] Crowder does not reference Park, but she uses similar imagery to describe how her son was "locked in his own private suit of armor," separated from her by an "impenetrable barrier" that "he had built around himself."[63]

With the help of a few months of intensive behavior therapy, the intact minds of all three children are recovered. Anne-Marie is six at the end of *Let Me Hear Your Voice* and has completely lost her diagnosis; her brother, at not quite four years old, has achieved age-appropriate functioning. Although he still engages in "brief episodes of excited hand flapping," their specialist discharges both children as requiring no further intervention or surveillance. Maurice, relieved, is now able to "savor [Anne-Marie and Michel's] childhood, a childhood redeemed."[64] Crowder, in contrast, didn't write her book until her son was grown, so is able to provide a longer view. "Today, Drew is twenty-one years old, and a student at a state university," she reports. And the book concludes with what becomes in this genre a common way of confirming recovery: an afterword by the previously autistic child, which often includes academic accomplishments and future plans, as well as gratitude for the parents' faith and labor. As Drew writes, "The most important instruction one can impart to the parent of an autistic child is 'Never give up.' "[65]

These books were followed by others advocating more alternative interventions, such as sensory integration,[66] the "floor time" model of child-directed play therapy,[67] diet and supplements,[68] facilitated communication,[69] and even horseback riding and shamanistic healing.[70] Some parents used a multipronged approach, combining what often seem like philosophically opposed treatments. Portia Iversen, cofounder of Cure Autism Now, for example, was an early champion of genetic research, which she advanced by raising funds, connecting researchers, and building AGRE (the Autism Genetic Resource Exchange), the largest private collection of genetic material from families with multiple autistic children[71]—a journey she describes in *Strange Son*, as well as her use of facilitated communication, a scientifically discredited technique. Marcia Hinds relied first on biomedical treatments to reduce the yeast overgrowth and brain inflammation that Bernard Rimland hypothesized were causal factors in autism, then turned to ABA, a strictly behavioral protocol.[72] And Susan Levin lists no less than twenty-one interventions she used with her son Ben over the course of six years, including the Son-Rise program created by Barry and Samahria (formerly Suzi) Kaufman, weekly vitamin B_{12} shots, intravenous immunoglobulin, craniosacral therapy, chlorine dioxide (a compound similar to bleach), daily enemas, and others.[73]

But no matter how different the strategies, these memoirs all share a similar rhetorical and narrative progression. Initially, the children are described as profoundly affected, displaying rages so violent, Levin admits, "our entire world revolved around avoiding Ben's tantrums,"[74] while Isaacson simply sums up, "Our lives *were* tantrum. Tantrum and the spaces in between."[75] Other disruptive and even dangerous symptoms include aggression, self-injury, and elopement—the compulsion to run away from a safe space, suffered by almost half of autistic children[76]—so persistent that Hinds reflects, "If Ryan were safe in a cage, I could take a break."[77]

But the most distressing symptom is the kids' unresponsiveness. Lori Ashley Taylor's daughter Hannah didn't "tur[n] her head when her name was called"[78]; Maurice's daughter Anne-Marie "wasn't seeing me at all. She was looking right through me!"[79]; Florance "felt more connected to my dog Coco . . . [who] was more responsive to me at six weeks than Whitney was at six weeks or six months."[80] Instead of interacting with their parents, the children spend their time "pull[ing] little pieces of string off the rugs or the furniture,"[81] "turn[ing] the miniature monster trucks upside down and spin[ning] the wheels for hours,"[82] or "turn[ing] the lights on and off a thousand times."[83]

And yet—despite their kids' minimal or absent language, their strange behavior, and their failure to meet developmental milestones, these parent-authors never doubt there is an intact mind in there, somewhere. Susan Levin describes her son Ben as "a child totally imprisoned in autism."[84] Cheri Florance titles one of her chapters, "An Intelligent Child Trapped Inside."[85] And Judy Barron remembers the conviction that kept her going, even though her son Sean's complete disconnection made him "a complete stranger to us": "There's a real child in there. . . . He's trapped and we've got to get him out."[86]

Maintaining this conviction, as Marcia Hinds notes, "in spite of all evidence to the contrary," is not easy. "During some of the more discouraging times, I just *hoped* [Ryan] was in there."[87] More than a quarter of a century earlier, Catherine Maurice had struggled with this as well: "I needed to think that there was still someone there, someone who would be there waiting as we fought our way through to her, someone, in fact, for whom all these tears were being shed." The passage in which Maurice describes her conflicted relationship with the intact mind is surprising and somewhat difficult to reconcile, given the arc of her story—which follows every step of this narrative even as she explains, "I never entirely trusted the psychoanalytic idea of a normal child locked with a chosen autism, and today I actively decry that notion and believe it has caused great harm." At the same time, however, she admits that this "construct, however fictional" of "the child imprisoned within, waiting to be reclaimed" is one that "parents who are going to fight for their child do need."[88]

Perhaps that's why even those memoirs in which the intact mind is not recovered use this imagery, as Josh Greenfeld did in *A Child Called Noah*. The labor of caring for severely autistic children, then teenagers, then adults, is intense and exhausting. It's extraordinarily hard to remain hopeful year after year when, as Bill Davis reports, "literally two or three hours almost every night were spent cleaning [feces]; getting stuff off the ceiling, disinfecting the room, changing the sheets, scrubbing his nails, and washing his hair"[89]; or, as Robert Hughes describes, you have to pick up your son at camp half an hour after dropping him off because he "took a bite out of his counselor's arm" and you lie awake at night wondering whether "he'd simply get harder to handle as the birthdays passed?"[90]

But these are decidedly not hopeless books. Hughes and Davis, while acknowledging their sons' challenging behaviors, celebrate their small accomplishments—by the end, Hughes' son Walker, at fifteen, can "read almost a full page from a Harry Potter book," although he "can't tie his shoes or point,"[91] and Davis's son Chris, still in diapers at six years old, "works the VCR like a pro."[92] It's their faith in their child's intact mind that allows both fathers to interpret these developments as "small vivid reminders of how near the Regular Kid actually was,"[93] as Hughes puts it—which, in turn, fuels expansive views of the future. "All agree that no one can set a limit to how far [Walker] can go,"[94] he concludes, while Davis's elaboration of his thought process in those moments is, for me, one of the most heartbreaking passages in any of the autism parent memoirs I've read:

> It's eerie because I see that child in there. And it saddens me because I think, "That's my little boy in there. There he is. I had him for a minute!" You want to reach out and grab him; just savor the moment. But it's gone. He's gone. . . . But it's an uplifting moment too because I know he's in there, and maybe in a few more years he'll reappear for good.[95]

Other parent-authors were under no such illusions, but they represent a decisive minority. Charlotte Moore notes, "A common belief among people not deeply familiar with autism is that there is a normal child trapped inside, struggling to get out. That's a false belief. I reiterate that Sam has no 'normal' core."[96] And Whitney Ellenby frames her 2017 memoir as a corrective to "public discourse on autism," which she finds "saturated with confusion and false hope" because of the " 'miraculous breakthrough' myth."[97] It speaks to the pervasiveness of the intact mind that these authors felt compelled to engage with this concept, even though it didn't reflect their own experience with their children. Agrees disability scholar Stuart Murray, "This central idea here of a space that is 'somewhere behind,' or of being 'locked in' . . . is, of course, a virtual orthodoxy in narrative depictions of autism."[98]

* * *

All of which begs the question: With so many memoirs documenting its recovery, isn't the intact mind in autism real? If not, what other explanation is there for so many dramatic transformations?

Let's start by eliminating some possibilities: I am not suggesting that these parent-authors are fabricating their stories or being deliberately deceptive in any way. I believe their description of their kids' concerning symptoms, from disengagement to lack of language to bizarre or violent behaviors, and I believe those symptoms largely resolved over time. In other words, I believe these books were written in good faith. I completely understand the need to share with other suffering families the intervention that you believe saved your child—I have felt it myself. My first book was about the tremendous success we had using electroconvulsive therapy (ECT) to drastically reduce Jonah's aggressive and self-injurious rages, which were so dangerous he was hospitalized for ten months when he was only nine years old.[99]

One theory that is often circulated is that the children weren't really autistic in the first place. Autism has always been diagnosed subjectively, based on checklists and observations by parents and doctors—there is still, today, no blood test or other biomarker for the disorder. In fact, it was the unreliability of the fourth edition of the *Diagnostic and Statistical Manual of Mental Disorders* (DSM-IV) subgroups of Asperger's, autistic disorder, and PDD-NOS (pervasive developmental disorder, not otherwise specified)—a 2012 study found that the labels children received depended not on their scores on standard assessments, but on where they were diagnosed[100]—that catalyzed the subsumption of these disparate categories into one, autism spectrum disorder, in the fifth edition, DSM-5.

But virtually all the parent-authors whose memoirs described the recovery of the intact mind are very defensive about this possibility—with the exception of Cheri Florance who, as mentioned earlier, argued that her son was not autistic and suffered instead from a previously unidentified syndrome she named after herself. Much more common is Judy Barron's afterword to the second printing of her 1992 memoir, in which she describes her initial assumption that researchers would have tremendous interest in her recovered son, and how wrong she was: "What we heard [from experts], however, was denial: 'If he recovered, then he never was autistic,'" a position she dismisses as evidence of the "territorial" nature of the field, which demands "a vested interest in [professionals'] own system and . . . rigid adherence to their methods."[101]

Other parent-authors rely on surrogates to confirm their children's diagnoses. Carol Johnson and Julia Crowder include a foreword by the giant of behavioral therapy himself, Ole Ivar Lovaas, to respond to such speculation. "The question may be raised whether Drew was in fact 'autistic,'" he writes. "Perhaps he was misdiagnosed and that Julia's story really is a misleading story in the sense that Drew would have gotten better without treatment. . . .

I will emphatically answer such a charge by stating that, according to Drew's independent diagnosis and our own observations, Drew fulfilled all the criteria of one having autism."[102] Marcia Hinds's memoir, in contrast, opens with a more emotional appeal by her recovered son, Ryan: "I don't want anyone to question the things my mom said in this book. Some will say I never really had autism or maybe that I was only mildly affected. I wish that were true."[103] And sometimes the debate raged outside the boundaries of the book—most notably, in the case of Jenny McCarthy, who released a statement in 2014 angrily refuting "stories circulating online, claiming that I said my son Evan may not have autism after all" as "blatantly inaccurate and completely ridiculous. Evan was diagnosed with autism by the Autism Evaluation Clinic at the UCLA Neuropsychiatric Hospital and was confirmed by the State of California."[104]

The fact is that researchers have known for more than fifty years that some children lose their autism diagnoses. For Michael Rutter, publishing in 1970, the phenomenon was very rare, with 1.5% adults achieving normal functioning.[105] In 2008, however, Molly Helt and her colleagues reviewed outcome studies and found that the number might be as high as 25%.[106] A more recent paper, which appeared in 2014, split the difference, reporting recovery in 9% of autistic children.[107]

Despite this large range, researchers' descriptions of recovered children share important similarities. Most importantly, all had IQs in the normal range as toddlers, whereas not one of the children with both intellectual disability and autism lost his or her diagnosis. And researchers freely admit that they cannot explain why some of the cognitively able children recovered completely while others didn't. The review by Helt and her colleagues found that "none of the studies found significant treatment differences between the children who moved off the spectrum and those who did not."[108] Another study that looked specifically at intervention history in autistic children with "optimal outcomes" was able to rule out what didn't work—diets and supplements—but when it came to teasing out efficacious therapies, investigators concluded that "neither particular types of intervention nor the number of hours of early intervention is sufficient to predict outcome."[109] To sum up: the children described in these memoirs may well have recovered, but it likely had little if nothing to do with the particular regimens espoused by their parents. They were just lucky.

Parent-authors don't see it that way, as previously discussed, proposing instead strict causal relationships between their children's specific treatments and their astonishing improvements. What goes unsaid in these accounts, however, is how they implicitly recapitulate the parent-blaming rhetoric of the psychoanalytic era that they so explicitly reject. Sociologist Amy Sousa argues that the common depiction of parents in contemporary memoirs of intellectual disability as "warrior-heroes"—so called because they "wag[e] battle against social and political forces to gain medical and educational interventions for their children despite the high personal and financial costs to themselves and their families"—"reflects a cultural shift in maternal responsibility from causing intellectual disabilities to curing them."[110] Jenny McCarthy, for example, describes the two types of mothers she sees at her son's preschool: "The 'woe is me' moms were talking about how they didn't get to shop or go to the beach with their friends anymore, and the 'I'll try anything if it will help my kid recover' moms were trading success stories about the latest treatments. I couldn't understand why *all* the mommies would not be up for something that *could possibly* help their kids."[111] Other memoirists were more direct about what was at stake, placing the responsibility for whether children recovered squarely on their parents' shoulders. "If anybody can help a child it's the parents," Bill Davis writes (somewhat aspirationally, it turns out, as at the end of the book his son Chris is still profoundly affected). "I can send my child to any school and follow any philosophy, but *I* must be keyed in to him for these things to work. It's a twenty-four hour a day commitment."[112] Susan Levin cannot emphasize the point enough, leaning heavily on italics to impress upon her readers, "*No one else can help your child the way you can . . . you* are the one who can help him recover."[113]

Just as Catherine Maurice considered the "harm" done by intact mind narratives even as her memoir followed the same arc, Lori Ashley Taylor pauses to acknowledge the impact of the cure burden that her own daughter's story perpetuates: "Parents hear about monumental improvements in individual cases and begin the treadmill of therapies in hopes that their child will have similar results. If he doesn't, they feel as if they haven't tried hard enough and that there must be another therapy that will be their magic bullet."[114] And that is exactly what we do, and how we think. I don't know any severely autistic children whose intact minds were recovered, but I know so many parents, myself included, who spent years in a state of ceaseless panic. How could I live with myself, I countered every time the rational part of my brain cringed at each new alternative treatment, if—and you can fill in the blank, auditory integration treatment, vitamin injections, hyperbaric oxygen therapy, etc.—turned out to be the one thing that could have tapped Jonah's intact mind, but I never tried it?

* * *

It seems appropriate, in closing this history of the intact mind, to return to where we started—to Clara Claiborne Park, who published a second memoir in 2001 called *Exiting Nirvana: A Daughter's Life with Autism*. Her daughter Jessy was no longer an eight-year-old girl, but a forty-three-year-old woman. I can't help but read *Exiting Nirvana* as a deliberate corrective to the intact mind narrative that originated in *The Siege*; Park opens the book by noting that Jessy's story "has not been about a miraculous recovery, though selective narration could give that illusion."[115]

To me, Jessy's accomplishments as enumerated in this second volume seem extraordinary, things Jonah will never do: for the past twenty years, she has worked full-time in the Williams College mail room; she cares for her elderly parents; she has become a well-known artist whose paintings have been featured in books and gallery exhibitions. Admits Park, "Who wouldn't hear, behind those words, others: 'miracle,' 'recovery,' 'cure'?"[116]

But the overwhelming message of *Exiting Nirvana* is that, while Jessy has made much progress, particularly in language and social awareness, she remains significantly disabled. Gone are the references to sieges and breakthroughs and walls. Instead we are told that Jessy will never be able to live independently, that she cannot work without supervision. That she still struggles with "the limitations of autism . . . [including] strange hypersensitivities, strange obsessions, strange compulsions, strange, explosive reactions."[117] At other points, Park's assessment is more encompassing: "You don't have to hear Jessy say more than a few words to know that you're not talking to a normal person"[118]—rather, she emphasizes, her daughter's mind "was severely limited."[119] One might even say, "impaired."

But most people don't read *Exiting Nirvana*; it was *The Siege* that the Autism History Project dubbed "still [one of the] most important parent memoirs about autism;"[120] *The Siege* that Marga Vicedo called "a bible for parents of autistic children, who continued, generation after generation, to rediscover the book."[121] And it was the concept of the "siege"—the fight to free the intact mind—that persisted in autism discourse, rather than the much gentler metaphor of a "journey" that Park adopted instead in *Exiting Nirvana*. It didn't matter that this understanding of autism was not consonant with prevailing medical theories about the disorder, or that most autistic children did not experience the transformational breakthroughs described in these memoirs. Regardless, "these ideas now form the currency of much public debate on autism," as Stuart Murray has observed.[122]

Ideas, debate, metaphors, concepts, discourse—the first half of this book has focused entirely on language. What words do we use to describe people with intellectual and developmental disabilities, such as autism? A completely reasonable response to these chapters might be, "OK, sure, perhaps our cultural descriptions of autism are a tad . . . euphemistic. But what's so bad about that?" Especially when it's what so many stakeholders in the community seem to want. In his memoir *Reasonable People* (which will be discussed in more detail in Chapter 6), Ralph Savarese describes his wife Emily's response to a cautionary note by researcher Lorna Wing about the limited skills of many autistic children: " 'What good does it do anyone to listen to it? What might hope endanger?' "[123] Autistic adults in the Neurodiversity movement have reacted similarly to depictions of autism they consider unfavorable, both in blog posts slamming "negative stereotypes about autism and autistic people"[124] and editorials published in prominent professional journals advising researchers and clinicians not to use words like "disorder," "severe," or "challenging behavior" because they "could be harmful to autistic people's well-being."[125]

I have made no secret of my issues with much Neurodiversity rhetoric, but I do agree that language has material impacts on the lives of autistic people (as it does for all of us) and that *harm* is an appropriate metric. The following case studies illustrate not only how the intact mind has come to inform much contemporary American policy and practice affecting the intellectually and developmentally disabled, but the very substantial harms that have accrued to the most cognitively impaired as a result—including the erosion of necessary supports and the proliferation of dangerous, pseudoscientific interventions.

PART II
THE CASE STUDIES

4
The Fight to Eliminate 14(c)

In the waning hours of the Minnesota state legislature's June 2021 session, a few brief lines were slipped into a 300-plus page omnibus bill. Although this was in clear violation of parliamentary procedure—the proposal never had a hearing in the senate, as required—and few representatives realized it had been added, the bill was signed by the governor, and the Task Force on Eliminating Subminimum Wage was created. Section 14(c) of the 1938 Fair Labor Standards Act authorizes certificate holders to pay employees—typically individuals with significant intellectual and developmental disabilities or psychiatric disorders—wages commensurate with their productivity. Unless the bill is amended, such sheltered workshops,[1] as they are often called, will be shuttered by 2025.

Minnesota has the largest number of 14(c) certificates in the country;[2] 6,000 adults earn a subminimum wage at programs operated by nonprofit agencies across the state.[3] One of those providers, Laura Johnson, the executive director of the Hubbard County Developmental Achievement Center, encouraged by the inclusion of 14(c) employers on the Task Force, accessed the application from the Department of Human Services website. She was stunned to find what can only be described as an ideological purity test she would have to check in order to be considered: "I understand the purpose of this task force is to develop a plan and make recommendations to phase out payment of subminimum wages to people with disabilities on or before Aug. 1, 2025. If selected, my role will be to support this purpose. This task force will not consider whether or not Minnesota should eliminate subminimum wages." No spots were set aside for current 14(c) participants or their family members, those most impacted by the closures.

Although the fluid status of 14(c) in the state makes Minnesota a compelling case study, this represents an important national issue. Eliminating 14(c) has been a key plank of the Disability Rights agenda for decades. Vermont, Maine, New Hampshire, and Rhode Island have already closed their programs; Alaska, Maryland, Oregon, and Texas are in the process of doing so.[4] At the federal level, Senators Bob Casey from Pennsylvania and Steve Daines from Montana introduced the Transformation to Competitive

Integrated Employment Act (TCIEA) in November 2021, which would phase out subminimum wage employment over five years. Much of the TCIEA was included in President Joe Biden's proposed Build Back Better bill—although in lieu of an outright ban, this legislation would provide $300 million to states that disavowed the practice. As of this writing, none of these bills has passed.

Yet, as committed as some disability advocates and policymakers are to abolishing 14(c), participants and their families are fighting to preserve it. In 2020, the U.S. Commission on Civil Rights (UCCR) released its Statutory Enforcement Report, "Subminimum Wages: Impacts on the Civil Rights of People with Disabilities." After recommending the elimination of 14(c), the Commission admitted that, not only had it received many more public comments than it had regarding any other issue, but that 98% of the more than 9,700 comments were in favor of preserving 14(c). Noted Commissioner Gail L. Heriot, in a dissent, "It would be difficult to find an issue for which comments were more lopsided."[5]

How to explain the stark contrast between the position of bureaucrats and disability advocates compared to that of many 14(c) employees and their families? It starts with the assumption of the intact mind, which informs the Commission's entire report. Quoted in this extensive document are experts like Jennifer Mathis, director of Policy and Legal Advocacy at the Bazelon Center for Mental Health Law, who stated, "Supported employment is founded on the belief that every person with a disability is capable of working competitively in the community if the right kind of job and the work environment can be found," as well as Julie Christensen, director of Policy and Advocacy at the Association of People Supporting Employment First, who "fundamentally question[s] the notion that someone simply cannot work competitively."

This sentiment is not unique to the UCCR report, but is foundational to the anti-14(c) lobby more broadly. Carol Glazer, president of the National Organization on Disability, calls the subminimum wage "immoral" because "people with disabilities are more than capable" and will "succeed . . . when given the chance."[6] Mississippi Congressman Gregg Harper agrees that "segregated, subminimum wage work is just an expression of low expectations that instills a false sense of incapacity in individuals who could become competitively employed with the proper training and support."[7] And the core assumption of Employment First—a framework developed by the Office of Disability Employment Policy at the U.S. Department of Labor and adopted by thirty-eight states—is "that all individuals, including those individuals with the most significant disabilities, are capable of full participation in Competitive Integrated Employment (CIE)."[8]

Nowhere in this narrative is there any acknowledgment of the profound cognitive and behavioral impairments that often afflict the intellectually and developmentally disabled—such as the violent rages, compulsive food stealing, and need for constant supervision described in some of the parent comments submitted to the UCCR. This notable omission motivated dissenting Commission member Peter N. Kirsanow to object that "this report is unmoored from reality in ways too numerous to count."[9]

* * *

In January 2022, I visited three Minnesota agencies that offer 14(c) employment and spoke with intellectually disabled participants, their parents, and administrators—all strong supporters of preserving this option. I did not seek out anyone who was dissatisfied with it—not because I'm denying that there are workshop employees fighting for more challenging, better-compensated jobs in the community, but because those voices are already privileged in the subminimum wage debate. In its 2011 report, "Segregated and Exploited: The Failure of the Disability Service System to Provide Quality Work," for example, the National Disability Rights Network (DRN) featured the story of a "young woman, in her 20s, who happened to have a cognitive disability," who was forced to give up her job in a college cafeteria—which she loved—for a placement in a "sheltered workshop," in which "she reported being very unhappy due to the boredom and repetitive nature of the work."[10] Even more shocking is the testimony in the U.S. Commission on Civil Rights Report from blind attorney Derek Manners: "My current salary, not to brag, is $250,000 a year. My sub-minimum wage hourly rate was $2.25 an hour. I've had the same level of vision in that job and in my current job."[11]

Although the first sheltered workshop in the United States was started at the Perkins Institute for the Blind in 1838, it should be noted that this population is rarely served in such settings now. After focusing on the blind and physically disabled for the first half of the twentieth century, workshops post-1950 increasingly catered to the intellectually and developmentally disabled, as parent groups in particular began organizing such facilities to support their children.[12] Today almost 85% of 14(c) participants represent this demographic.[13]

This is not at all to minimize the impact of Manners's story—or that of the unnamed cafeteria worker, for that matter. But this debate is not about whether all disabled adults should be forced into workshops—it's about whether all disabled adults should be forced out of them. Over the past decade, the number of 14(c) certificate holders has dropped by two-thirds in the United States,[14] at least partially due to an increased emphasis on supporting the disabled in integrated employment—a development rightly celebrated by stakeholders on both sides of this debate. Lori Schluttenhofer, vice president of Day and Employment Services at Opportunity Partners, the largest agency I visited, remembered, "When I started in this field thirty years ago, when a student left transition services, the thought was, what center do I want to go to? Now so many more are considering advanced education or community placements." This one model, however, "will never work for everyone"[15]—an argument raised by virtually every one of my interlocutors. As policymakers at both the state and federal level push to completely eliminate 14(c) regardless, I chose to focus on those who would be most affected by such a decision—those whose voices (or, perhaps more importantly, whose silences) challenge the dominant narrative around this issue.

My first visit was to the Hubbard County Developmental Achievement Center (DAC), a small agency in Park Rapids, Minnesota, that serves seventy-two clients with a range of cognitive impairments and psychiatric disorders. Like all the facilities I visited, the DAC offers multiple program options; fewer than half of their participants hold subminimum wage jobs. And some clients make minimum wage or even higher, depending on the work they're doing at any particular moment. Lisa K.,[16] age thirty, for example, earns minimum wage when she weaves rugs sold in stores owned by the DAC, because after years of practice that began with simply ripping strips of fabric, then rolling them into balls used by the weavers, then operating the loom itself, she has become very adept at this labor. But when she works in the DAC thrift store pricing and shelving donated items—tasks she does accurately, but very slowly—she makes less.

At the DAC main building, I observed clients engaged in different jobs. One person manned a shredder—all the programs I visited have shredding contracts with local businesses, as this job requires few skills—but almost every other project involved making crafts to sell at the three DAC stores: rugs, birdhouses, and fire-starters (compressed bricks of sawdust and candle wax used in fireplaces). A fully equipped gym was unused while I was there, and sign-up sheets on the bulletin board offering a range of activities, including swimming, pickleball, and music, had few signatures. "I usually prefer to work," Lisa explained in her thin, high-pitched voice.

The DAC opened in 1945 and serves clients across a forty-mile radius of largely rural Hubbard County, in the northwest part of the state. Before a placement opened up at a group home near the DAC main building in Park Rapids, Lisa's parents spent seven years driving fifty miles roundtrip, twice a day, just so she could meet the DAC van to take her the rest of the way. The dearth of appropriate services and the logistical issues posed by the DAC's vast catchment represent unique challenges that the larger, Twin Cities–based agencies I visited don't face. "The state is pushing everyone into community jobs," Executive Director Laura Johnson said. "But half the stores in town are closed from January through May. And even the shops that are open have just one full-time employee working retail."[17] The DAC has had to be creative, opening three stores to provide employment opportunities: an antique shop, a depot that sells used appliances, furniture, and building materials—both of which are staffed exclusively by higher functioning clients earning minimum wage or higher—and the thrift store, Bearly Used, its most successful business. One of the frustrating parts of this debate is that, although Bearly Used is located right on Park Rapids' main street, and serves as a hub—not only for its disabled employees but for seniors and other locals who meet every week to chat and check out the new merchandise—the state does not consider it integrated employment, simply because it is owned by the DAC.

Considering how to spin off the stores into their own nonprofit enterprises is just one of the ways Johnson is planning for the elimination of 14(c), in case she and the thousands of affected participants, family members, and providers are unable to derail the plan set in motion last June. "We're not going to close, not on my watch," Johnson stated. She has been busy writing grants to fund expanded community-based activities, like art and theater, determined not to leave her clients stuck at home. "But if we lose that work option, it's going to be very painful for participants who have been doing this for decades, some for thirty years or more."

Certainly Lisa would be disappointed. "I love my jobs," she explained. "I want to work until I'm at least seventy." She so clearly articulated the sense of independence that working at the DAC gave her—and how sad she was at the temporary loss of that independence, when she had to return to her parents' home during COVID, which made her eyes "all wet and weepy"—that she seemed to me perfectly capable of holding a competitive, integrated position. But her mother, Debbie, explained that Lisa, who is autistic, also suffers from severe obsessive-compulsive disorder (OCD) and anxiety that can provoke very challenging behaviors.

"Lisa develops odd obsessions, like drinking out of every water fountain she sees, or blowing out every table candle she sees—awful if you are at a restaurant with candles," Debbie elaborated. "And some pose real safety risks, such as her need to touch the side of every teapot or kettle she sees, just to make sure it is hot. The most dangerous is her compulsion to open the car door if she hears the beep to remind you to put on your seatbelt. She has opened her door on the freeway going over sixty miles an hour! We are very careful about setting the child locks on our car, and reminding her group home staff that this is an absolute necessity."

But worst of all are the aggressive episodes that can occur when Lisa gets, as her mother describes it, "stuck."

"I get upset and anxious easily when people get into my workspace or unexpected things happen," Lisa agreed. Once, when she was having trouble with her loom, she angrily took a scissor to the warp—the strings across the loom that provide the base for the weaving—which took an entire day to repair. Other times, she has physically attacked her support staff, fellow participants at the DAC, and other residents at her group home. "I live in fear that Lisa will do something so violent she gets kicked out," Debbie said. "If she were booted out, where would she go?"

The high rate of challenging behavior among the intellectually and developmentally disabled is largely unacknowledged by anti-14(c) advocates who insist that everyone with a disability can hold competitive, integrated employment. A 2006 Canadian study found that almost 52% of over three thousand subjects—clients at three rehabilitation agencies in Quebec—engaged in violent behavior over the course of a year, including self-injurious and aggressive episodes, as well as property destruction.[18] These results are remarkably consistent with those of a 2013 study that looked at autistic children enrolled in the United States–based Autism Treatment Network and found that 53% were physically aggressive.[19] The severity of these outbursts varies across the population—in the most extreme cases, autistic individuals have blinded or concussed themselves from repeatedly hitting themselves in the head, or left their caregivers with bruises and broken bones—but the vast majority of employers obviously and necessarily have a zero-tolerance policy for such behaviors.

"Lisa's not even five feet tall, but she's left big bruises on my husband and myself," Debbie told me. "The staff at the DAC know her so well, they can really help redirect her when she gets agitated. She needs that level of support all the time. Providing that in a competitive workplace, where the staff-to-client ratio would be much smaller—probably one-to-one if she were the only disabled employee—would be financially unsustainable when job coaches are typically paid $40 an hour."

Eddie K., also thirty, has a similar history of dangerous behavior. Autistic, intellectually disabled, and nonverbal, he frequently left his mother bitten and bleeding, the walls of his house covered in holes. Once he threw a TV out the window; another time he bolted out of the house and was hit by a car (thankfully, he was uninjured). By the time Eddie was sixteen, his parents Carl and Gail could no longer safely manage these behaviors, and he moved to a group home. But once he graduated from school, no day program would accept Eddie until Merrick, Inc., took a chance on him in 2018.

Merrick is a medium-sized nonprofit that opened in 1964 and now operates three locations serving approximately 340 intellectually and developmentally disabled clients. Like the Hubbard County DAC, Merrick runs several different programs, including a life enrichment program that offers horticulture, pet therapy, music, art, and theater to those who have no interest in work; facility-based employment; competitive employment; and mobile crews that fulfill contracts with various commercial partners, such as local grocery stores or medical centers.

I visited Merrick's largest location, a 52,000-square-foot facility in St. Paul. The setup of each part of the building reflected the diverse needs of the work done there. Instead of the DAC's single office shredder, Merrick has an entire shredding room, with three industrial-sized machines each taller than a person, as well as two balers to pack the shreds. "The challenge is to break down these processes into smaller steps so that clients can get paid for some part of a job and be a valued member of the team," Executive Director John Wayne Barker explained to me.[20]

In another room, clients sat at workstations assembling products for which they receive a piece rate: some slipped greeting cards into plastic sleeves (the Merrick team processes about 60,000 cards per week); others assembled COVID test kits; still others packaged bicycle tools. Eddie, his father told me, could never sit still long enough for one of these positions. Instead, he is part of a four-person crew that goes out with a job coach to pick up plastic from various sites. "Eddie loves being active," Carl said. "He loves riding in the truck and loading the plastic." Once they return to Merrick, other participants operate the machinery that bales the plastic, before loading it onto trucks and sending it to its final destination, where the material is repurposed as composite decking. "That's one million pounds of plastic that otherwise would have ended up in a landfill," Barker said.

I asked Carl how he knew that Eddie liked working at Merrick, since he can't answer the question directly. "His problematic behaviors have diminished so much now that he is happy," Carl answered. "Eddie used to have a one-to-one aide, but he doesn't need it anymore." He paused. "I'd like to say it's miraculous that he can be on a one-to-four crew at Merrick, but that's not right—it's been hard work by people who know how to give him choices, how to redirect him."

My final site visit was to Opportunity Partners, which was founded in 1953 and is now the largest 14(c) provider in Minnesota. Their primary location can serve over 400 people, but I went to a smaller facility outside Minneapolis to meet Alex S., age thirty, who has worked there for the past six years. Although opponents often dismiss 14(c) employment as "busy work,"[21] the project Alex was working on—packaging medical supplies—was considered so vital to national security that when the program was briefly closed during the pandemic, staff members had to come back from furlough to do the work themselves.

Just like the Hubbard County DAC and Merrick, 14(c) represents only one of the programs that Opportunity Partners offers. Approximately 270 out of the 1,200 intellectually and developmentally disabled clients hold subminimum wage positions; others make minimum wage, while some opt to earn no wages at an enrichment program. Besides the work floor, Opportunity Partners also has enclave teams that go out with job coaches to various community locations, such as universities or local businesses, where they perform a range of jobs, including cleaning, assembly, and packaging. "We had a number of people prior to COVID who not only had an independent community job, but they also worked on a supported employment team, and came back here to work on the floor or take enrichment classes," Lori Schluttenhofer told me. "It's a misconception that it's either/or. Often community jobs are part-time only. A lot of people are served best by a combination of services."

Mindy S., Alex's mother, has wondered whether her son could advance to the point that he could be as productive as a nondisabled peer. Alex doesn't engage in the challenging behaviors that Lisa and Eddie do, but he is autistic and intellectually disabled—although he is also what's known as a "calendar savant," someone who can tell you what day of the week any particular date from the past or future did or will fall on—and requires round-the-clock supervision. "It would have to be a job that's very repetitive, and there would have to be a lot of focus on that, and it would take years. I'm not sure how someone who is at the third-grade level gets employment," she mused. But that goal hasn't been prioritized because, most importantly, "Alex loves where he is. When he comes home, all he talks about is going back to his work center on Monday. He can't stop talking about '51st Avenue' [what he calls Opportunity Partners, since that's the address], that's all he talks about."

Alex is not nearly as conversant as Lisa, but he did answer my questions. He told me what he was working on, and when I asked him if he liked working at Opportunity Partners, he told me that yes, he did.

"A lot or a little?" I asked.

"A lot," he said, so softly I could barely hear him over the indiscriminate buzz of people working and the sound of "Old Time Rock and Roll" playing over speakers set into the ceiling.

* * *

I asked Johnson, Barker, and Schluttenhofer what their agencies would do if 14(c) is eliminated in August 2025, as the Minnesota bill requires. All three are looking to expand their other offerings, but that largely involves increasing activities that now fall under the category of enrichment: art, music, and community outings like bowling or petting cats at the animal shelter. Not one anticipates significant migration into competitive, integrated employment, although the entire movement to abolish the subminimum wage hinges on this outcome.

The fact is, as the UCCR freely acknowledges, "there is [*sic*] no national data available that tracks what happens to people with disabilities who were working for 14(c) certificate holders in states that have abolished the payment of subminimum wages"[22]—despite the fact that twenty years have passed since Vermont closed its 14(c) programs, so theoretically it would not have been difficult to track those outcomes. "It's as if they don't really want to know," Barker observed.

The limited studies that have been done actually suggest the opposite. A 2012 update from Washington state noted that, despite an investment of $50 million into employment services for the intellectually and developmentally disabled, only 17% of severely affected adults were able to find jobs.[23] A 2015 George Washington University analysis of the impact of closing sheltered workshops in Maine reported that, post closure, individuals with intellectual and developmental disabilities only worked an average of twelve hours per week, the fewest in the country, while utilization of non-employment day services (what some parent commenters to the UCCR dismissed as "glorified babysitting"[24]) increased by almost 500%.[25] A longitudinal study published the same year examined the vocational experiences of more than 200 adults with various levels of intellectual disability in Oklahoma between 1994 and 2009, and found that, while participation in sheltered workshops dropped by about two-thirds over this fifteen-year period, there was no corresponding increase in integrated employment—although the number of subjects who were sitting at home almost tripled.[26] Anecdotally, the UCCR report included testimony from a U.S. representative from Wisconsin concerning an agency in his state that had served 500 disabled clients before giving up its 14(c) certificate, after which it was only able to support 65[27]—which was very similar to a story repeated to me by several of my interlocutors about a big Minnesota agency that also decided to move away from 14(c), certain that the imminent abolishment of this option was a fait accompli, leaving about a thousand clients without services.

Not only are the promises of 14(c) opponents completely lacking in empirical support, but their attacks against this service model reflect both a deep misunderstanding of how it works today and why it appeals to so many intellectually and developmentally disabled adults and their families. The Minnesota programs I visited have waiting lists up to hundreds of people long; Merrick's John Wayne Barker told me, "If I could build another floor on this building, I could fill it with people who want 14(c) work."

It is hard to reconcile that with the DRN's 2011 report on subminimum wage employment, whose title "Segregated and Exploited" (reiterated in their 2012 follow-up, "*Beyond* Segregated and Exploited" [emphasis in original]) basically sums up the two main arguments that advocates use to galvanize opposition to 14(c). The UCCR report makes similar accusations of financial exploitation, describing participants earning an average of $53.44 per week while "providers and associated businesses . . . profit from their labor."[28] This implication that employers are getting rich off the backs of disabled employees—foregrounded in the accompanying letter to President Donald Trump, Vice President Mike Pence, and Speaker of the House Nancy Pelosi—seems disingenuous, given that the Commissioners go on to report just a few pages later that, as of January 1, 2020, 93% of certificate holders were nonprofit community rehabilitation programs, and only 2% were for-profit businesses.[29] Not only is 14(c) not a lucrative enterprise—"a savvy business person would never get into 14(c)," Lori Schluttenhofer acknowledged—but these programs often lose money that must be recouped elsewhere. Opportunity Partners, for example, relies in part on fundraising, while the Hubbard County DAC operates three stores that generate $700,000 in revenue per year. "We'd never make it without those," Executive Director Laura Johnson told me.

But there's a larger reason the financial exploitation argument is, despite its prominence, a red herring in the 14(c) debate: at the three Minnesota agencies I visited, not one subminimum wage employee is expected to live off what he or she earns—which is the typical case for this service model. Participants' paychecks often represent just a tiny fraction of the government support they receive, which may include direct cash in the form of Supplemental Security Income (SSI), as well as funding for residential services, healthcare, transportation, leisure activities, and placement at the 14(c) facility itself. Ninety percent of Merrick's clients, for example, receive such packages. The budget of one participant I met was approximately $120,000/year, while another was over $160,000. And the wages this latter young man made at his 14(c) program—only about $3,000 in 2021, as he is severely impaired—were deducted from his SSI, creating what his father described as "a zero-sum game"—meaning that his total budget remained stable no matter how much he earned.

Not only have opponents completely misrepresented the economics of 14(c) by repeatedly describing it as a "life of perpetual poverty,"[30] but their romanticization of minimum wage labor—or, as the DRN refers to it, the "dream"[31]—is notably discordant with other scholarship that portrays it as a life of precarity. Most famously, activist Barbara Ehrenreich pursued three-month-long stints working in unskilled positions, including waitressing, housecleaning, and sales, which she described in her 2001 book *Nickel and Dimed: On (Not) Getting by in America.* Rather than the "choice," "self-determination," and "meaning" that the DRN conflates with minimum-wage employment,[32] Ehrenreich describes coworkers trapped in "invisible and even disgusting" jobs (often more than one) they were forced to take to support their families. As she concludes her series of experiments, "No one ever said that you could work hard—harder even than you ever thought possible—and still find yourself sinking ever deeper into poverty and debt."[33]

More fundamentally, the DRN's explicit goal of transforming the disabled into "active, tax-paying member[s] of the community"[34] perpetuates a surprisingly neoliberal hierarchy of value that has been roundly critiqued across the academy. Neoliberalism—the valuing of citizens according to their ability to participate in free markets—is very similar conceptually to what historian Michelle Murphy has called "the economization of life," which "names the practices that differentially value and govern life in terms of their ability to contribute to the gross domestic product."[35] Murphy's lens is not disability, but race; she examines discourses and practices of population control mainly in Bangladesh, which she finds motivated by purely economic concerns. But is there any population more "surplus and aggregate" than the intellectually and developmentally disabled, more devalued and marginalized? Murphy couldn't ask for a better example of how the economization of life is deployed to "divide life into categories of more and less worthy of living"[36] than the utter contempt with which disability advocates dismiss 14(c) participants: "Someone compensated to the tune of a few cents an hour is hardly employed," sniffed Autistic Self-Advocacy Network founder Ari Ne'eman hyperbolically, in a blog post arguing for the elimination of 14(c).[37]

Or maybe it's not that surprising. As historian Sarah Rose has argued, "access to paid work has long served as the foundation of social and economic citizenship in the United States." For Rose, disability was "invented" in the decades following the Civil War, as industrialization created the demand for a standardized labor force that excluded those whose diverse impairments were more easily accommodated in rural communities. This new association of disability with economic dependency and lack of productivity was highly stigmatizing, contributing to the warehousing of this population in custodial institutions.[38]

Some of the earliest organized disability advocacy crystallized around this fight against employment discrimination. The League of the Physically

Handicapped formed in 1935 to protest the exclusion of most disabled applicants from Works Progress Administration (WPA) jobs, and after a well-publicized occupation of the WPA's Washington, D.C., offices, successfully secured an audience with head Harry Hopkins.[39] Importantly, League members did not contest the connection between work and value; rather, with slogans such as "We Don't Want Tin Cups. We Want Jobs" and "We Are Lame But We Can Work," they asserted their capabilities and challenged stereotypes that excluded them from the workforce.[40] Workshops run by private charities were explicitly targeted in the League's "Thesis on Conditions of Physically Handicapped"—submitted both to Hopkins and President Franklin D. Roosevelt—as sites "engaged in shameful exploitation of the physically handicapped."[41]

More than fifty years later, historian and polio survivor Paul Longmore famously burned his first book in front of the Federal Building in Los Angeles to protest work disincentives that threatened Social Security recipients with the loss of their benefits if they accumulated more than $1,800 in assets. Since many, like Longmore, relied on these benefits to pay for support staff to assist in activities of daily living as well as for expensive, life-sustaining technologies (Longmore used a ventilator), the practical result of this policy was to preclude the disabled from pursuing meaningful employment. For Longmore, his biography of George Washington symbolized the culmination of his academic aspirations. "My book represents, not just my work, but the work that we all want to do and could do," Longmore announced before igniting it on October 18, 1988. "We want access to work. We want access to the American Dream."[42]

More recently, Rose notes, scholars of women's and labor history have begun to disentangle ideas of citizenship from standards of economic productivity. Other critiques have emerged from disability studies: Jasbir Puar, for example, offers a similar argument to Murphy's, noting that the "incorporation of certain disabilities into neoliberal economic circuits . . . ultimately serves to further marginalize and exclude most people with disabilities."[43] In turn, Puar cites the work of disability scholars David Mitchell and Sharon Snyder, who criticize the stratification of disabled people by how closely they fit "reigning concepts of normalcy" and coined the term "able-disabled" to describe "those disabled people who . . . gain entrance into late capitalist cultures . . . but leave the vast majority of disabled people behind."[44] And yet, despite this consensus rejection of capitalist definitions of human value, scholars have largely let go unchallenged what even a non-academic like UCCR Commissioner Peter Kirsanow could recognize as the persistent "conflat[ion of] 'productive' with 'worth' "[45] by anti-14(c) advocates.

Because, ultimately, the debate over 14(c) really isn't about money—it's about that other claim in the DRN's reports, *segregated*. The Disability Rights Movement and the allied Neurodiversity Movement are hegemonically opposed to *all* disability-specific settings—like specialized classrooms or schools, larger residential facilities (such as intentional communities, campuses, and farmsteads), and 14(c) vocational programs. As long as misrepresentations about the economics of subminimum wage employment and discordant celebrations of capitalist paradigms are used to attack such "institutional" programs, most academics have been content to let them slide.

The origin of this attitude is not hard to decipher. For almost a hundred years, many Americans with intellectual and developmental disabilities were institutionalized in facilities that grew in some cases to confine thousands of residents. With inadequate funding—the Willowbrook State School, for example, had a 1-to-40 staff-to-patient ratio—abuse and neglect were rampant. Geraldo Rivera, whose 1972 exposé ultimately led to the closure of the facility, described it as "a crime against humanity," in which severely intellectually disabled children were left "lying on the floor naked and smeared with their own feces."[46]

The world of vocational services has its own Willowbrook, which 14(c) opponents use to anchor all discussions of subminimum wage employment: the notorious Henry's Turkey Service, which virtually enslaved a thousand intellectually and developmentally disabled men in Iowa over the course of thirty years, forcing them to engage in gruesome work (such as eviscerating turkeys with their bare hands) for $65 per month, while being housed in a rodent- and trash-infested converted schoolhouse. In 2013, a jury awarded an unprecedented $240 million to the disabled employees.[47]

To be clear, the intellectually and developmentally disabled represent an extraordinarily vulnerable demographic that has experienced abuse and neglect across every setting—from institutions to the family home, from workshops to community-based employers. A 2013 British study of employees with learning, psychological, or emotional disabilities, for example, reported that "the likelihood of experiencing any ill-treatment at work was increased by 177%," including the staggering fact that these employees were almost nine times more likely to have been physically attacked at work than their nondisabled coworkers.[48] There's no doubt that significant oversight is required over all programs that serve this population.

And 14(c) programs are subject to robust oversight. Large agencies like Opportunity Partners have staff members whose sole job is to ensure compliance with Department of Labor regulations, which include regular audits and unannounced site visits. Wages are not subjectively determined by employers, but are calculated using a strict formula that compares a participant's pace in a particular job to that of the average nondisabled pace (calculated by taking the mean of timed trials by three different nondisabled workers), while also considering prevailing rates for that labor. For example, if three nondisabled employees can assemble 100 widgets in an hour, and are paid $15/hour, a 14(c) participant who completes 25 widgets in the same time period would earn $3.75/hr. Every six months, that participant would be reassessed to see if his or her productivity had increased, and rates adjusted accordingly. Many employees at the 14(c) programs I visited in Minnesota end up making minimum wage or higher as they become more skilled at their jobs.

None of this matters to inclusion advocates, who routinely conflate all 14(c) programs with Henry's Turkey Service—and all congregate care facilities with Willowbrook—and argue that disability-specific settings are, by definition, "isolating" and, as we've seen, "segregating." They cite the Americans with Disabilities Act and the 1999 Supreme Court *Olmstead* decision as "inclusion mandates"[49] that require disabled individuals to receive services solely in integrated settings.

But even a cursory reading reveals that this is a gross misinterpretation of *Olmstead*. The majority did find that the plaintiffs, Lois Curtis and Elaine Wilson, had the right to receive services in the community rather than in a Georgia state institution. But the justices did not issue a blanket decree. Supports should be provided in the community, they argued, under three conditions: that community services are appropriate, desired by the individual, and can reasonably be provided by the state. And the justices clearly recognized how many people did not fit these criteria. In a concurring opinion, Justice Anthony Kennedy warned, "It would be unreasonable, it would be a tragic event, then, were the Americans with Disabilities Act of 1990 to be interpreted so that States had some incentive, for fear of litigation, to drive those in need of medical care and treatment out of appropriate care and into settings with too little assistance and supervision."[50]

The blind spot informing persistent misinterpretations of *Olmstead* seems to be that inclusion advocates simply cannot imagine why anyone would choose a disability-specific setting—even though this has never been a consensus position across the broad disability community. One of the earliest and most prominent leaders of the Disability Rights Movement, polio survivor Judy Heumann, fondly recalled the warmth and connection she experienced at a summer camp just for disabled kids, where campers who felt self-conscious and excluded among their nondisabled classmates during the school year had the opportunity to dance, date, and share their similar experiences.[51]

Of course, the largest faction of the disability community to actively oppose inclusion is the deaf, who have been fighting since the ascendancy of oralism at the end of the nineteenth century to preserve a culture articulated, in the United States, through American Sign Language (ASL). Rather than the limited success deaf children typically achieve communicating exclusively by speech and lip-reading, deaf novelist Sara Nović argues for ASL instruction as the pathway to rich and diverse expression—including poetry, video, and plays—in a 2017 essay bluntly titled, "The Hearing World Must Stop Forcing Deaf Culture to Assimilate."[52] In a more academic take, Australian scholars Jan Branson and Don Miller characterize the mainstreaming of deaf students as "epistemic violence."[53]

But instead of acknowledging that not everyone—disabled or not—shares the same hierarchy of values or definition of quality of life, the UCCR report, as Commissioner Peter Kirsanow critiques, "elevates 'inclusion' and 'integration' over every other concern."[54] For some people with intellectual and developmental disabilities, holding competitive, integrated employment may very well be extraordinarily important—and they should, without question, receive whatever supports necessary to succeed. But my interlocutors had other priorities that they believed were best met in their—or their children's—14(c) programs.

As discussed earlier, one common reason motivating such placement was that participants' cognitive impairments and behavioral challenges precluded competitive, integrated employment. This extended beyond the actual skills required to execute any particular job, to the more general ability—or even desire—to comport to the expectations of employers. Debbie K., for example, explained that one of the reasons her daughter Lisa is much less productive at the thrift store is that she's easily distracted—she starts pricing books, then ends up reading them. This was not an unusual story. The administrators I spoke with all told me that no one is ever forced to work, and that participants often decide to spend extensive periods chatting with their friends instead.

This type of behavior would simply not be tolerated by conventional employers—who, Barbara Ehrenreich reports, try to extract every second of labor out of every day. At Wal-Mart, pausing to even briefly converse with fellow employees is considered "time theft"; at The Maids, she notes, "We do not walk to the cars with our buckets full of cleaning fluids and utensils in the morning, we run, and when we pull up to a house, we run with our buckets to the door."[55]

These employers also do not, as Opportunity Partners does, set up a haunted house room for their employees on Halloween, or take them on rides in classic cars. Nor do they break up the workday by inviting them to participate in play readings, like the Hubbard County DAC does. Given the more congenial pace, the extracurricular activities, and the lack of necessity (since, as mentioned earlier, costs of living are typically covered by other government benefits), it's not surprising that, as Lori Schluttenhofer reports, clients sometimes choose to give up integrated job placements to return to Opportunity Partners. "We had one autistic young man who, after working on the work floor for several years, got a job at a Pot Belly sandwich shop," she recounted. "The manager adored Sam and was committed to keeping him employed. But Sam didn't like it, he kept ditching work. Eventually he came back because he needed his relationships."[56]

Most fundamentally, that's what the debate over all disability-specific settings, including 14(c) programs, comes down to: different definitions of community. Peter Kirsanow was struck by the UCCR's guiding assumption "that it is preferable to spend time among those without disabilities than among those with disabilities,"[57] but that's only because, I presume, he hasn't read much Neurodiversity literature. As a coalition of organizations, including the Autistic Self-Advocacy Network (ASAN), Self-Advocates Becoming Empowered (SABE), and the National Youth Leadership Network defined it in a position paper, "community must 'integrate with people who don't have disabilities, and this does not mean staff.' "[58] In other words, a group of intellectually and developmentally disabled people is segregated, isolated, and institutional *by definition*. The goal of disability policy thus becomes to embed the disabled person with as many nondisabled people as possible—a somewhat ironic finding from a summit comprised *solely* of twenty-five "self-advocates with developmental and intellectual disabilities."[59]

Debbie K. understands this attitude well, as she once held a similar view. "I'm a teacher, and I was always very pro-integration," she told me. "I knew the laws for special ed, and I made sure Lisa was included in typical classes with a one-on-one para [aide] all through school." As her daughter's graduation neared, Debbie toured adult programs with trepidation. "I was very apprehensive," she said. "I didn't want to see Lisa stuck in one of those workshops, I had that mindset. But when I actually visited, I saw people working there who just loved it."

It wasn't long after Lisa started at the DAC that Debbie and her husband Marc saw a side of their daughter they had never seen before. They had always thought that Lisa was shy, because she made no friends in school. "But after one year at the DAC, we saw more social growth in her than in her entire integrated school career," Debbie added. "Turns out, Lisa is extremely social, *with her peers*—people who don't mind when she recites the scripts from the last four *Arthur* episodes, or imitates something that one of the characters did in a

Madeline video. We went to a DAC picnic and she was running around visiting with everyone." Now, the former inclusion advocate argues that describing the DAC as segregated "devalues disabled people" because it suggests that the cognitively impaired "only count if they're surrounded by the nondisabled."

Certainly for Lisa K., her disabled coworkers represent one of the things she likes best about working at the Hubbard County DAC: "Many of my coworkers have become my friends. A lot of them have disabilities just like I do, like Down syndrome. We have so much in common. My one friend likes princesses just like I do." Although Eddie K. can't articulate how he feels, his father Carl told me that Eddie "recognizes whether people like him or not, so if people are uncomfortable or ignore him, he acts out." He attributes Eddie's improved behavior, in part, to the fact that staff and fellow participants at Merrick "engage with him, talk to him, even though he can't talk back. He likes being noticed and engaged." Alex S., like many individuals with severe autism, is less interested in his peers than in staff members, but he is tremendously attached to his job coach, who has worked with him since he first started at Opportunity Partners.

As for the parents, they didn't think the government should be in the business of legitimating certain communities over others, and were frustrated at the persistent denigration of their children's preferred communities just because they primarily comprised individuals with intellectual and developmental disabilities. "No, Lisa doesn't want to be the one disabled employee at Wal-Mart working among a nondisabled workforce," Debbie K. said. "I think a lot of the folks at the DAC feel the same way."

Data from Merrick, Inc., confirms this preference. The 2016 Workforce Innovation and Opportunity Act (WIOA) requires that state vocational rehabilitation agencies annually conduct a Career Counseling and Information Referral (CCIR) session with each person in a 14(c) program, to present the advantages of competitive, integrated employment. "Last year, 204 clients went through a CCIR session," John Wayne Barker reported. "And 198 said they did not want to pursue minimum wage work. That's 97%."

"Lisa absolutely prefers to be surrounded by peers," Debbie added. "I'm not sure why that's so difficult to understand."

* * *

Even if the supporters of 14(c) I met in Minnesota successfully amend the June 2021 bill and win the battle, they have already lost the proverbial war. State regulations that took effect on January 1, 2021, substantially limit accessibility to 14(c) programs. No one under twenty-five years of age is allowed to earn a subminimum wage, and three failed community-based placements are required before a 14(c) program can even be considered. Of even greater concern to families is the 36-month limit now placed on these positions. "The presumption is that if you provide the right training, people can move to competitive employment," Barker explained to me. "As you know, that's a myth for some who have chronic, lifelong disabilities. If they can't, the only alternative is life enrichment services." Or sitting at home, which is what Hubbard County DAC Executive Director Laura Johnson describes as a "common situation" for the high school graduates who had participated in her agency's programs through their schools but no longer qualify.

Lisa K., Eddie K., and Alex S. are all grandfathered in, so the three-year limit doesn't affect them. But I couldn't help thinking of Mindy S.'s dismissal of enrichment as an appropriate setting for Alex: "I don't want him sitting around coloring all day."

It's hard to imagine that's what Disability Rights advocates want for him either. But one of the most surprising things about this debate is how little opponents are willing to discuss modifying 14(c), rather than eliminating it. "If we're concerned about people being diverted, let's have a conversation about it," Opportunity Partner's Lori Schluttenhofer proposed. "From my perspective, we're doing a much better job now supporting people who want to work in the community." She acknowledged, however, there was still work to do: "If there are people getting stuck, maybe we need a better way of screening them out and helping them make the transition to competitive employment. But let's make sure the people who really need 14(c) can access it." The most common aphorism I heard, from multiple interlocutors, was, "Don't throw the baby out with the bathwater."

Perhaps a better slogan would be, "Nothing about us without us." It's already been claimed by Neurodiversity proponents, and Disability Rights advocates more broadly, to assert the rights of the disabled to participate in the decisions that affect their lives. But what the 14(c) debate exposes is how exclusive that "us" really is. For some reason I'll never understand, Lisa, Eddie and Alex don't count as "us." Neither do the 97% of Merrick's clients who went through the CCIR process, nor the 98% of the 9,700 commenters to the UCCR who supported the preservation of 14(c).

Notably, those left out are the most severely cognitively impaired, and the family members who support them. "The state of Minnesota has, over the past thirteen years, intentionally made it more difficult to provide onsite services to people with chronic and severe disabilities," John Wayne Barker told me. "The people who are hurt when 14(c) closes are those with the most significant barriers to employment," Schluttenhofer agreed. "We're not hanging on to this because it's easy, because it's not. We're not hanging on to it because we make a big profit, because we don't. 14(c) is not our mission, it is a tool for us to provide that mission. Our mission is to enhance the lives of people with disabilities."

It's a difficult mission, since not everyone's lives can be enhanced in the same way. In a disability service provision landscape allegedly driven by the vision of "person-centered planning," my interlocutors were mystified and frustrated by the push to force everyone with intellectual and developmental disabilities into one model. The spectrum of impairment in this population is impossibly broad, including college-educated self-advocates like Derek Manners and Ari Ne'eman and nonverbal, cognitively impaired adults like Alex S. and Eddie K., who don't understand the concept of the money they earn, never mind why the amount is so controversial. It seems completely obvious to supporters of 14(c) that we need a similarly broad range of supports to reflect such diverse needs and preferences. As Lisa K. explained to me, "Handicapped people should have the right to choose where they work and who they work with, just like all people should get to choose who they love and the jobs they have and where they live."

5
The Erosion of Guardianship

The discourse around guardianship is just as enflamed as that around 14(c), if not more so. This court-appointed model of substitute decision-making for incapacitated adults has been described as a "civil death"[1] analogous to "eugenics."[2] At the United Nation's World Autism Awareness Day in March 2017, Chair of the Committee on the Rights of Persons with Disabilities Theresia Degener demanded that guardianship "must be repealed," casting it as gross a violation of human rights as "slavery" and "genital mutilation."[3]

Many of the stakeholders leading the battle against guardianship are the same neurodiversity organizations fighting not only to eliminate 14(c), as discussed in the previous chapter, but also to expand facilitated communication, the subject of the next one—including the National Disability Rights Network, the Arc of the United States, the Autistic Self Advocacy Network (ASAN), and TASH (The Association for the Severely Handicapped). As I was writing this in early 2022, a 2020 video recirculated through my social media that nicely illustrates this synergy: produced by the Self Advocacy Resource and Technical Assistance Center (SARTAC)—an affiliate of both ASAN and TASH—it featured a severely autistic, nonverbal young man, John McCarty, who terminated his guardianship (which was described as "heart wrenching and degrading") after establishing his capabilities and articulating his preferences through the Rapid Prompting Method, a form of facilitated communication.[4]

And this alliance seems to be accumulating the same legislative and regulatory successes against guardianship as it has against 14(c) programs. On January 1, 2022, Washington became the latest state—joining Texas, Delaware, Alaska, Wisconsin, Indiana, Nevada, Colorado, North Dakota, Louisiana, Rhode Island, and the District of Columbia[5]—to pass a law requiring that supported decision-making, or SDM (a less restrictive but importantly less accountable model than guardianship, as will be elaborated below), be considered or, in some cases, actually pursued before guardianship.

So I assumed I would have little difficulty recruiting interlocutors to speak on the consequences of this erosion of guardianship for adults with autism and other intellectual and developmental disabilities. I disseminated a request for subjects through the same channels I used to procure my 14(c) interviews: autism organizations, like the National Council on Severe Autism (NCSA), Facebook groups for parents of autistic children. But whereas I had more volunteers than I could use for my chapter on the sub-minimum wage, few people reported adverse outcomes from their guardianship hearings. In fact, not once did I hear a story that I had expected to hear many times: *We went to court, and the judge denied guardianship*. Instead, I frequently heard the opposite. "I was nervous but the judge was very friendly," Tracy C. recalled about her 2018 hearing in Florida. "He talked, or should I say tried to talk to my son. . . . We were done probably in about an hour." Kate R. was moved to tears by the judge's compassion at her son's hearing in Maryland two years later: "He wished us luck, and told us we were really good parents."

"Our guardianship hearing was fabulous! The judge was kind and attentive," agreed Michigan mother Abby P., who was awarded guardianship of her son in 2018. "When it was almost over, the judge asked my son if he had anything to add, and he leaned into the microphone like he was testifying before Congress or something, and said 'that's a wrap, court is dismissed,' and the judge laughed out loud and told him, 'I get to say that!' "

Obviously, my reach is not universal; I make no claim that the experience I anticipated has never transpired. But still, as confirming examples failed to materialize, I had to wonder: why, in the specific case of guardianship, did there appear to be such a notable mismatch between the tenor of the discourse and the experience on the ground?

* * *

The history of guardianship extends back to the ancient world. In the fifth century BC, the Greek playwright Sophocles read from his most recent play to successfully establish his competence after his son pursued guardianship over him. And "tutors" were routinely charged by Roman courts with managing the property of those deemed incapable of doing so, such as spinsters, widows, and orphans.[6]

American guardianship law traces more directly back to the English *Statute De Prerogativa Regis*, a 1324 law based on *parens patriae* (literally, "parent of the country") that authorized the king to protect the property of those considered "unsound of mind."[7] These legal relationships were purely financially motivated, pursued by those seeking control over another's estate, and required mental competency hearings to confirm whether in fact the person in question was an "idiot"—that is, someone with lifelong and permanent impairments—as the Crown could not assume the property of those with temporary or episodic illnesses who might recover their capacities.[8] After the American Revolution, that *parens patriae* power fell to the states, which took different approaches to assessing competency. Some used county probate courts, while others borrowed from English tradition and established lunacy commissions.

Definitions of competency have unsurprisingly changed over time and have been greatly informed by societal values. In her analysis of guardianship hearings in Wisconsin from the 1860s–1940s, historian Kim Nielsen exposes the heteronormative expectations that made unmarried men and women especially prone to attempts by family members to take control of their estates via guardianship. Other common reasons for challenging competency included alcoholism, old age, and disability—factors that were considered impediments to reigning conceptions of economic productivity. What becomes clear in Nielsen's account is that guardianship centered more on the disposal of property than the provision of care until well into the twentieth century. Notably, she reports, African and Native Americans never instituted guardianship proceedings, largely because of their relatively impoverished status compared to the white landowners jockeying to consolidate their own financial interests at the expense of more vulnerable family members.[9] It was not until 1963 that John Kennedy's Task Force on Law of the President's Panel on Mental Retardation acknowledged that "in the past the law has seemed to place more emphasis on the protection of property rights of the retarded than on the protection of their personal rights" and called for a balance between these, as the members saw them, equally important commitments.[10]

This new concern for the rights of the intellectually disabled reflected not only Kennedy's personal investment as the brother of an affected sister, Rosemary, who had been lobotomized in 1941, but also the language of the nascent Disability Rights Movement—which Joseph Shapiro argues was launched the year before the Task Force was created, when post-polio quadriplegic Ed Roberts enrolled at the University of California at Berkeley. Roberts, who spent eighteen hours a day in an iron lung, had to fight to get Berkeley to admit him and California's Department of Rehabilitation to pay for his tuition, as well as the services he would need to matriculate. Ultimately, his success inspired others with similar disabilities to apply, and by 1967 there were a dozen paralyzed students living in the Berkeley infirmary that called themselves the "Rolling Quads." This group, guided by the principles of "Independence. Self-sufficiency. Mainstreaming. Disability as a social problem," would go on to start the Center for Independent Living in 1972. Notes Shapiro, "Roberts redefined independence as the control a disabled person had over his life. Independence was measured not by the tasks one could perform without assistance."[11] Or, as Roberts's colleague Judy Heumann would later phrase it, "Independent living is not doing things for yourself. It is being in control of how things are done."[12] Autonomy, in other words, has been a central plank of the Disability Rights Movement since its inception.

So it's no coincidence that the report of Kennedy's Task Force represents the earliest publication I've found that proposes the creation of limited guardianships that could be "carefully adapted to the specific requirements of the case." While complete, or "plenary" guardianships were indisputably required for intellectually disabled adults who were "judicially determined to be incapable of undertaking routine day-to-day decisions"—a determination that should not be arbitrarily made but that required "a comprehensive clinical evaluation covering medical, psychological, educational and social factors"—others might only need a guardian's help with a subset of decisions, such as those involving finances or healthcare. "We urge that, as far as possible, mentally retarded adults be allowed freedom," the Task Force advised.[13] This call for limited and individualized guardianships was echoed the following decade, by both the Commission on Mental Health, which was established by President Jimmy Carter in 1977, and the American Bar Association's Commission on the Mentally Disabled, which released a Model Guardianship Statute in 1978.[14]

Even as discourse shifted during this period—from descriptions of the intellectually and developmentally disabled as objects of pity or charity to a rights-based advocacy reflecting the influence of both the Women's and Civil Rights Movements—it's important to note exactly what rights stakeholders foregrounded in these conversations. The focus on limited guardianship clearly demonstrates a growing concern that guardianship as it was historically utilized represented a blunt instrument that frequently and unnecessarily disempowered cognitively impaired adults from making those decisions that they could make for themselves.

But other organizations were equally committed to ensuring that members of this vulnerable population were protected from potentially catastrophic outcomes they were utterly incapable of anticipating. And they also used the language of rights. In 1967, the Stockholm Symposium of the International League of Societies for the Mentally Handicapped stated, "A retarded person . . . who has a general inability to manage his life has a right to have a guardian who is legally and actually qualified to protect his interests and promote his personal welfare." The next year, the International League of Societies for the Mentally Handicapped issued its Declaration of General and Special Rights of the Mentally Retarded, which included a similar claim: "The mentally retarded person has a right to a qualified guardian when this is required to protect his personal well-being and interest."[15] And in 1971, the United Nations Declaration on the Rights of Mentally Retarded Persons affirmed that "[t]he mentally retarded person has a right to a qualified guardian when this is required to protect his personal wellbeing and interests."[16]

This tension between the rights to protection and self-determination crystallized in the 1970s around what minister and Disability Rights activist Robert Perske termed "the dignity of risk." Perske described how, during a research trip to Scandinavia, he had met intellectually and developmentally disabled adults who were taught to use public transportation independently, work dangerous equipment like drills and saws, and pursue romantic relationships. "We cannot continue the type of over-protection we usually give the mentally retarded in our country," he argued. "To deny any retarded person his fair share of risk experiences is to further cripple him for healthy living. Mentally retarded persons may, can, will, and should respond to risk with full human dignity and courage."[17]

The dignity of risk was quickly folded into the increasingly popular philosophy of service provision for the intellectually disabled known as "normalization." Articulated by Wolf Wolfensberger in 1969, adherents of this philosophy advocated for "utilization of means which are as culturally normative as possible, in order to establish and/or maintain personal behaviors and characteristics which are as culturally normative as possible."[18] In other words, supports for this population should be designed to resemble typical nondisabled life—including mainstreamed classes for children; small, integrated homes for adults; age-appropriate recreation; and standard schedules and types of employment. Taking risks and being allowed to fail are an important part of "normal" life, advocates argued, and should not be denied to the intellectually disabled.

But what kind of risks, and what kind of failures? Perske tells the following story:

> A severely retarded 10 year old named Billy, wandered away from an institution where he lived and became lost in the woods nearby. The temperature was below freezing. All off-duty personnel were called back to the institution to form emergency parties to search for the boy. Two moderately retarded teenage boys, Ray and Elmer, asked a staff member if they could search for Billy, too. The staff member "moved through channels," and after some time, received approval for the boys to join in the search. As it turned out, Ray and Elmer found the lost boy. The superintendent gave them special recognition and letters of commendation. As a result of this incident, the staff became more aware of the 75 other moderately retarded adolescents (boys and girls). These teenagers might have been mobilized

more efficiently and quickly than the staff had they not been denied their fair and prudent share of risk taking.[19]

Ray and Elmer were heroes. But critics of the dignity of risk were more concerned about the Billys of the world. Should Billy be allowed to make the decision to walk away from the institution, when he was so clearly incapable of understanding the risk to his life of getting lost overnight in the cold? In 1974, Canadian psychiatrist Darold Treffert coined his own phrase, "dying with their rights on," to describe how the "pendulum of history" had swung from "an attitude of stifling paternalism toward the mentally ill to the outright abandonment of their needs." Treffert wrote about psychiatric patients, not the intellectually disabled—as examples, he included an anorexic woman who starved to death after a judge refused to forcibly hospitalize her, as well as a college student who hanged herself after signing out of the ward she had been admitted to following an earlier suicide attempt—but his call to "protec[t] the right of both that patient and those around him or her from tragic and untoward effects of the patient's illness"[20] seems equally applicable to anyone whose judgment is significantly impaired.

To be fair, even the most strident advocates for normalization acknowledged that the dignity of risk allotted to the intellectually and developmentally disabled must be, as Perske qualified, "commensurate with their functioning."[21] And Treffert himself believed that "the right of the psychiatric patient to remain free" was "a precious and important right."[22] Advocates for the cognitively impaired may have disagreed about exactly where the "reasonable middle ground" fell between Treffert's two poles of "stifling paternalism" and "outright abandonment," but the need to balance appropriate care with individual autonomy remained a pervasive theme in this literature—until 2006, when the United Nations attempted to foreclose the entire debate with its Convention on the Rights of Persons with Disabilities (CRPD), which reversed the protections articulated in the Declaration on the Rights of Mentally Retarded Persons and asserted an absolute and universal competence: "Persons with disabilities enjoy legal capacity on an equal basis with others in all aspects of life."[23]

* * *

Concerns about the abuse of guardianship had been percolating for decades. In 1987, the Associated Press published its report on a year-long investigation that concluded that a system designed to be "a crucial last line of protection" was instead "failing many of those it is designed to protect." The AP study focused on guardianship of the elderly, but many of the violations it uncovered—including "little or no evidence of necessity" and the "fail[ure] to guard against abuse, theft and neglect"—read as indictments of the system as a whole. Reporters described judges who "rubber-stamped" applications for wards who were not even present, professional guardians who had legal responsibility for hundreds of wards *each*, family members who abandoned their elderly parents or grandparents after spending all their money, and nursing home and hospital administrators who disturbingly used guardianship "as a hedge against liability in tough decisions such as amputations and disconnecting life support systems." The subtitle of the report, "Declared 'Legally Dead' by a Troubled System," must have particularly resonated with advocates invested in asserting and defending the rights of the disabled.[24]

The AP report catalyzed an immediate and tremendous response. Within days, the U.S. House Select Committee on Aging convened a hearing. By the following year, the National Guardianship Association was founded (and would go on to issue a Model Code of Ethics in 1991), and the American Bar Association's Commission on the Mentally Disabled and the Commission on Legal Problems of the Elderly had issued over thirty recommendations for guardianship reform.[25] Over the next fifteen years, every state revisited their guardianship laws to some degree, from minor tweaks to wholesale revisions. These changes typically included stronger protections for proposed wards, more specific definitions of "incapacity," the use of limited guardianships, and increased court supervision.[26]

But the degree to which these reforms were actually implemented remained unknown. In 2004, the U.S. Government Accounting Office (GAO) surveyed courts across the country and found an uncoordinated system that kept little data on the number of individuals under guardianship or how—or even whether—those guardianships were monitored.[27] And a 2005 study funded by the Retirement Research Foundation similarly acknowledged that "statistics are scant," and could only hazard a guess at the number of adults under guardianship (about 1 out of every 1,750 Americans, according to an estimate that was almost a decade old), never mind saying anything meaningful about their outcomes.[28] Although exposés would periodically appear in the newspapers—like a 2003 article in *The Washington Post* that described guardians who profited while their demented or schizophrenic wards languished in homeless shelters or filthy group homes[29]—it was impossible to know the extent of these abuses. There was little evidence to discredit the decidedly ambivalent conclusion of a 1983 Penn State study, which found that, broadly considered, "guardianship in and of itself does not have significant positive impacts on the alleged incompetent, [but] neither are there many . . . horror stories."[30]

So Article 12 of the CRPD, according to an editorial in *Lancet Psychiatry*, represented a significant, and surprising, reversal "away from previous intergovernmental agreements and from what is currently deemed best medical practice."[31] Titled "Equal recognition before the law," this section not only affirmed that everyone with any kind of disability "enjoy[s] legal capacity on an equal basis with others in all aspects of life," as noted earlier, but required signing nations to "take appropriate measures to provide access by persons with disabilities to the support they may require in exercising their legal capacity," and even specified the right of all disabled citizens "to own or inherit property, to control their own financial affairs and to have equal access to bank loans, mortgages and other forms of financial credit."[32] If the intact mind assumption is not completely obvious in this position, legal scholars Gerard Quinn and Abigail Rekas-Rosalbo make it explicit, noting that the CRPD "amounts to a statement of faith that there is always some kernel of the 'self' discoverable in persons even with severe intellectual disabilities and that the focus of efforts should, henceforth, be on expanding our admittedly narrow repertoire of discovery techniques to uncover the 'self' lurking behind the disability."[33]

Over 180 nations have since ratified the CRPD, but by 2014 it was clear that "the implications [of Article 12] seem to have largely flown under the radar of most governments."[34] Not one signatory had taken the claim of universal capacity literally, interpreting it instead in the context of previous guardianship reform that had emphasized maximizing the autonomy of the intellectually and developmentally disabled as much as possible through the use of limited guardianships and supported decision models when appropriate. So the Committee on the Rights of Persons with Disabilities issued its first General Comment on the CRPD on Article 12, noting the "general misunderstanding of the exact scope of the obligations of States parties" and lamenting the "general failure to understand that the human rights-based model of disability implies a shift from the substitute decision-making paradigm to one that is based on supported decision-making." There was nothing aspirational about Article 12, the Committee emphasized. Signatories were obligated to immediately take steps to "abolish" *all* "substitute decision-making regimes such as guardianship, conservatorship and mental health laws that permit forced treatment."[35]

Comment No. 1 has been strongly criticized for what opponents describe as a bizarre and wholesale rejection of the material implications of severe cognitive impairment. Germany's statement that "the Committee's interpretation is not shared by the State Parties in general; not even by a substantial minority . . . Germany remains convinced that there are situations in which persons with disabilities simply are not able to make decisions even with the best support available" reflected the feedback of other nations, including Norway, Denmark, and France.[36] Other responses were less diplomatic. "The Committee has lost sight of reality here," scolded Dutch health law professor Joseph Dute.[37] Agreed the Law Society of Scotland, "One of the worst forms of discrimination against anyone with a disability is to fail to recognize and provide for the extent and consequences of their disabilities, and to pretend that these do not exist. . . . It is a fundamental breach of their human rights not to provide appropriate mechanisms to ensure that their interests are safeguarded and their rights exercised."[38] To date, only Peru, Costa Rica, and Colombia have passed the necessary legislative changes to bring them into compliance with Article 12.

* * *

The United States signed the CRPD in 2009 but has never ratified it.[39] This doesn't mean that guardianship laws have been unaffected by the United Nations' rhetoric. As noted earlier, several disability organizations have advocated for laws promoting supported decision-making as a precursor or alternative to guardianship, and a dozen states have passed such legislation.

But the definition of "supported decision-making" has remained murky and contingent since the term was coined by the Taskforce of the Canadian Association for Community Living in 1992.[40] As many scholars—even those supportive of SDM—have pointed out, the framework "is used in many different contexts, and it is often unclear exactly what people mean when they refer to it."[41] In its SDM toolkit, the Autistic Self-Advocacy Network defines this model as one that "gives people with disabilities the help they need to make choices about their lives," and goes on to add a key criterion: "The person with a disability chooses a person that helps with decisions . . . the supporter gives advice, but the person with a disability makes the final decision." Although this may be adequate for those with mild intellectual and developmental disabilities, nowhere in this guide does ASAN entertain the possibility that it is exactly the cognitive impairments that make a person a candidate for guardianship that preclude the thoughtful selection of advisors and the ultimate ability to exercise sound judgment.[42]

What concerns family members of more severely impacted adults the most is the complete absence of legal supervision or protections under SDM. As the Autism Society, San Francisco Bay Area, noted in a letter of opposition to a proposed bill in California, under SDM, "If the person with I/DD wishes to run outside naked, others must abide. If he wishes to eat nothing but Skittles for weeks at a time, others must abide. If he refuses medical care for a gaping wound, others must abide. If she wants to have sex with a felon who has stalked her online, others must abide. . . . If he wants to send his Special Needs Trust assets to hackers from North Korea, others must abide." On top of this are the very real fears of manipulation by so-called friends: "If he wants to sell a supporter or someone else his car or home for pennies on the dollar, others must abide."[43] And these are not just hypothetical situations. Rebecca J., one of my interlocutors, was stunned to discover that her nineteen-year-old autistic son, Tyler, had left the house with no money and no clothes to spend the weekend with a 40-year-old man from Wyoming who had flown 3,000 miles, rented a car, picked him up, and took him to a hotel. Rebecca called the police and they did bring him home, but because she doesn't have guardianship, the officers said "that he could make his own decisions—even if they were bad ones." They told her not to call them again if he disappears.

Abuses have, without question, also occurred under guardianship. One 2010 review from the GAO found that guardians stole or misappropriated more than $5 million from over 150 wards[44]—but reforms since the 1980s have repeatedly called for more court monitoring, not less. Notably, SDM proponents consistently fail to address why such exploitation won't occur even more under SDM arrangements that involve similar power disparities but no legal accountability whatsoever. Perhaps that's because there are no data to support such claims: scholarship on both sides of the SDM issue agree that the push for this legislation has occurred in the complete absence of empirical research demonstrating that SDM increases autonomy without, as Piers Gooding acknowledges in a book supportive of this model, "result[ing] in the unreasonable transfer of risk and uncertainty by the state to persons with disabilities."[45]

And yet, the SDM legislation continues to grow. As I write this in early 2022, bills are pending in Illinois, Kansas, Maine, New Hampshire, New York, and California—whose version is the most extreme and would require SDM to be tried with everyone, no matter how cognitively impaired, before guardianship could be attached. And if there's anything that illustrates how surreal this debate has become for the families of severely autistic and intellectually disabled adults, it's the poster child of the SDM movement in that state: pop star Britney Spears. In fact, an entire #FreeBritney movement has mobilized to overhaul conservatorship (what guardianship is called in California).

There is much tragedy in Spears's case. But I don't think anyone, regardless of position on guardianship, would support the stripping of someone's rights in a pro-forma, ten-minute hearing that the person in question wasn't even allowed to attend, or the seemingly punitive decisions by her father to deny her access to a cell phone or time with her own children while pocketing millions of dollars of her earnings.[46] More important for this debate, however, is that, while Spears may have been suffering from some mental health issues, she is a capable woman who, in the thirteen years she was under conservatorship, released four albums and grossed over $130 million on a global tour. As a frustrated Jill Escher, president of the National Council on Severe Autism, titled a 2021 blog post, "Earth to Disability Activists: The Britney Spears Conservatorship Is Irrelevant to Cases of Adults with Severe Autism."[47]

It's not just Britney that's irrelevant. The examples typically cited by guardianship critics highlight extremely atypical cases—such as a *Vice* exposé featuring an *attorney* whose mother filed for guardianship when she was a child to control an inheritance.[48] For Escher, the use of such cases to call for an end to all guardianships disingenuously shifts focus off the much more typical candidates for this model of substituted decision-making—cognitively impaired adults like her son Jonny, who is "nonverbal with a measurable IQ in the 20s, and with functional skills of a preschooler."[49]

Or like Leslie F.'s twenty-one-year-old son Nick, who suffered a disfiguring injury because of Massachusetts regulations intended to protect individuals from unnecessary interventions. Nick and his twin brother Elliott are both severely autistic and suffer from aggressive behavior that necessitated their placement in residential schools when they were eleven and twelve years old, respectively. As they approached their eighteenth birthday in 2018, Leslie filed for guardianship. Elliott, nonverbal and incontinent, had been assessed at the functioning level of a three-year-old, and although Nick had some simple words it was obvious that neither of her sons could make important decisions for themselves.

Elliott's guardianship was granted immediately, but because Nick had been prescribed a small dose of the antipsychotic Abilify to reduce his violent behavior, he required what in Massachusetts is called a Rogers guardianship. According to the state website, this grants permission for guardians to approve " 'extraordinary' medical treatment"[50]—although the use of antipsychotics in this population is not at all extraordinary. In fact, Abilify and the related antipsychotic Risperdal are the only drugs that have been approved by the FDA to treat self-injurious and aggressive behaviors frequently associated with autism. Approximately 20% of autistic kids and more than 40% of autistic adults have taken them.[51]

"Nick's Rogers guardian was essentially opposed to anti-psychotic medication—I found out later she had a brother who was under a Rogers guardianship—and fought me tooth and nail without ever having met my son," Leslie explained. Although she had been granted a temporary guardianship, the court-appointed attorney kept filing to have the guardianship rescinded—a fight she took to the Massachusetts Supreme Court, although Leslie was never informed of that hearing. "The Supreme Court took my guardianship away, and sent it back to the probate court saying that they had received a well-written letter from Nick saying that he didn't want me to be his guardian. But he could never have written anything like that."

Importantly, Leslie felt the original probate judge was "trying to bend over backwards to be kind." He pressed the Rogers guardian about why she had never met with Nick, and in April 2019 restored the temporary guardianship. But while Leslie was waiting for the paperwork to arrive in the mail, Nick lost a tooth after biting his teacher's arm, and the dental hospital refused to treat him without proof of guardianship. By the time his staff took him to Boston Children's Hospital, it was too late to save the tooth. And that wasn't all the family lost. Leslie, a single mother, was fired after missing too much work for all the court dates. The process to date has cost her thousands of dollars. And she lives in fear that if Nick's antipsychotic medication needs to be increased—which seems likely, as he has become more self-injurious, including leaping off his bed headfirst onto a concrete floor—that the Rogers guardian will fight to stop it.

This story—of the legislative and regulatory obstacles to guardianship that parents encountered before they ever entered a courtroom—is a common one. "Tennessee has made conservatorship inaccessible for a lot of families," Jane K. told me, describing her battle to obtain conservatorship for her eighteen-year-old daughter Jocelyn, who suffers from severe autism, intellectual disability, epilepsy, and other medical complications as the result of a rare genetic condition, SynGap1. "You can't file until the day your child turns eighteen, so there's no way to enter adulthood protected."

Jane had grave fears over what might happen to her daughter while her paperwork wound its way through the system. "It takes sixty days to file a petition for conservatorship—that's sixty days of an incapacitated adult being left vulnerable to anyone coercing them into anything they want," she explained. And it didn't take long for that to happen. "Jocelyn's teacher said she could no longer communicate with me without Jocelyn's permission," Jane said. "The teacher called to let me know—with Jocelyn's permission, allegedly—that the school had scheduled a meeting to discuss implementing restraint and isolation, and that Jocelyn had signed agreement to this plan. But that didn't make any sense—the school had previously determined that Jocelyn needed a decision-maker in all areas, she has an estimated IQ of 47." Jane felt she had no choice but to pull Jocelyn out of school.

There was another option—an emergency conservatorship, which would cost $3,500 but only took four days for a temporary order. Jane, also a single mother, did not have that kind of money. But her daughter's exposure without the conservatorship was significant. Not only was Jane concerned about exploitation, but she had real fears about what might happen if Jocelyn—whose rages are so violent that Jane locks herself in her bedroom to keep her daughter from hurting her—was involved in a police interaction. "If she hit or kick an officer—which she would do because she doesn't care who it is—and there were no conservatorship in place, she would be taken to the county jail and charged with assault on a police officer. We don't have a mental health option in our county. Imagine: Jocelyn going to jail! That was a serious, serious concern for me." Ultimately, Jane took out a loan to pay for the emergency conservatorship.

Similar to Leslie F.'s experience, once Jane got into the courtroom, the judge was very supportive. "Jocelyn was an uncontested case with a notarized affidavit from the highly respected Vanderbilt Complex Care physicians and the unquestioning backing of both her guardian ad litem and attorney ad litem," she recounted. "It was an easy, innocuous process."

* * *

How to explain why, even as states increase the legislative and regulatory burdens on families seeking guardianship over their autistic and intellectually disabled children, parents consistently report meeting little resistance once they actually get in front of a judge? I suspect the answer lies in the necessary and personal interaction that comprises a guardianship hearing. Bills to promote the use of SDM—or, for that matter, to eliminate 14(c) programs—are proposed and voted on at the most abstract level, by advocates and policymakers who may have never met a single person with severe cognitive impairment. It sounds progressive and empowering to celebrate the autonomy of disabled adults by freeing them from supports painted as oppressive, outdated, and paternalistic, such as guardianship and sheltered workshops. And when the only disabled individuals consulted are those who would never want or need such services, of course that vision—so much easier than the reality of adults who will require a lifetime of specialized, expensive, around-the-clock care to keep them from hurting themselves or others—is likely to prevail.

But, face to face with a Jocelyn, or a Nick, or a Jonny, and buried in the extensive documentation of their intellectual disabilities, minimal communication skills, and profoundly dangerous behaviors, no judge is likely to deny guardianship, regardless of her ideological commitments. The risk of significant harm is just too self-evident, the implicit responsibility too great.

This observation suggests a possible intervention as state and federal governments target the intensive, disability-specific services that severely autistic and intellectually disabled individuals often require to maximize their quality of life. What if, before defunding or eliminating any educational, vocational, and residential settings, policymakers were forced to spend even a short amount of time with those who rely on such models and their families—to sit with my twenty-four-year-old son Jonah, for example, while he sucks his thumb and watches the same thirty-second clip of *Elmo's World* over and over, to observe the swelling of cauliflower ear where he hits himself in the head, to listen to me enumerate our greatest and most hard-fought victories: toileting, shoes, haircuts, plugging in his iPad when it dies instead of throwing it out the window of a moving vehicle? Could they really walk away from that experience completely unaffected?

Perhaps this sounds idealistic and impractical, but it would not be particularly difficult to implement. Consider that there are, according to most recent estimates, currently about 1.3 million Americans living under guardianship[52]—which required about 1.3 million individual meetings between judges, incapacitated persons (when possible; occasionally, due to acute medical and/or behavioral challenges, the presence of the person is waived), and their families. In contrast, there are fewer than 7,400 state representatives in the entire country. Even if each and every legislator met with a severely autistic and intellectually disabled adult and his or her family, that would still represent a tiny fraction of the meetings involved in establishing all those guardianships. Adding in the unelected officials who typically run state disability agencies would admittedly increase that number, but there's no reason this engagement couldn't be facilitated in small groups, rather than one-on-one.

And I've seen this kind of exposure really change people. In January 2016, I presented to the Interagency Autism Coordinating Committee (IACC)—which advises NIH on how to spend its autism research budget—about the need for a broad range of housing options to meet the very diverse needs of the autistic population. Afterward, prominent autistic self-advocate and IACC member John Elder Robison approached me and said that he thought that autistic adults should decide for themselves where to live. I agreed that they should whenever possible, but that Jonah's cognitive impairments precluded such complex decision-making.

John was skeptical. As he recounted in a *Psychology Today* blog about our conversation, "I had a hard time believing that. My dogs can pick which place they want to sleep, and they are non verbal with pretty low IQ."[53]

Later, he would apologize for such a dehumanizing analogy. But reflecting on it after I recovered from my shock, I realized that his response revealed another assumption that informs proposals to restrict or eliminate guardianship: that important choices, like where to live, are easy and natural. In fact, they only appear seamless. Disability researchers Karrie Shogren, Michael Wehmeyer, and their colleagues offer a definition for decision-making that emphasizes prerequisite abilities to assign probabilities and anticipate consequences: "the act of choosing among competing courses of action based on an understanding of the probable outcomes of those courses of action. This necessitates an understanding that multiple factors influence the decision making process."[54]

Jonah can, technically, choose between two options. He wouldn't understand abstract words like "live" or "move," but if he were familiar enough with the places, I could ask him, "Jonah, do you want to go to place A or place B?" and he would pick one. But the more impactful the decision, the more the reasons matter. Jonah would not consider the staff-to-resident ratio, the training of the direct care staff, the range of activities, or the level of crisis support. He wouldn't care about cleanliness, or abuse records, or financial viability—really, any of the criteria that would be important to me and Andy. Instead, his selection might reflect differential access to peanut butter, the color of Gatorade in the refrigerator, or, most likely, the order of presentation. Jonah almost always picks the first alternative he is offered—unless he very strongly favors the second, in which case he will make us rephrase the question: "Place B or Place A, WHICH ONE?"

Standing in the IACC meeting during the fifteen-minute break between sessions, I couldn't explain all of this to John Robison. Instead, I just asked him to come meet Jonah—a response to those who perpetuate relentlessly positive depictions of the disorder that writer and autism parent Hannah Brown calls "the Autism Challenge": "spend an hour, just one hour, taking care of a low-functioning person with autism."[55] John wasn't the only person I invited, but in 2019 he became the first person to take me up on it.

Our meeting was facilitated by John Donvan and Caren Zucker, authors of the 2017 autism history *In a Different Key* and producers of a documentary of the same name. John and Caren had asked my family to represent the severe end of the spectrum in the film, and, after reading about my previous interaction with John Robison, decided to fly him in from Boston to spend a day with our family. Because he doesn't know the scripts—"number one IS"; "I'll be right back"; "fun list"—Jonah didn't speak with him much. But they engaged nonverbally, with Jonah hanging on John's arm as we walked around our neighbor's field, enjoying the lovely spring weather. Afterward, I asked

John if he still felt like I had misrepresented Jonah's cognitive abilities. "No, I can't talk to Jonah about where he wants to live," John acknowledged. "And I understand seeing Jonah when you say that your conversations about where Jonah wants to live are very limited also." John was still committed to maximizing self-advocacy for those on the autistic spectrum, he emphasized to me. "But I also understand that there is a point on the disability continuum where the disabled person has only a limited ability to participate. And our obligation to protect those people is always with us."[56]

It was such a productive discussion, I was surprised to find out, months later, that it had been completely cut from the movie. John Donvan called to give me the news. He and Caren, steeped in autism politics through their research, writing, and lived experience (Caren also has an autistic son), had brought me, John Robison, and Jonah together because they anticipated that our interaction would be powerful and generative—and they believed that it was both of those things. But when they showed the scenes to focus groups unconnected to the autism community, they were met with bewilderment. Jonah's profound impairments were immediately apparent. Why was his lack of capacity so contested? Clearly, he could not make important decisions for himself, and obviously, as his parents, Andy and I were most qualified to fill that role. "We would have had to spend too much time contextualizing the issue," John explained. I could tell from his tone that he was afraid I would be disappointed, and I was for a moment, until I realized that the focus group response couldn't have been more encouraging for the future of the guardianship debate. "For the rest of the world," he elaborated, "it's just common sense."

6
The Resurgence of Facilitated Communication

Nothing is more predicated on the intact mind than facilitated communication (FC). Imported from Australia in 1989 by Syracuse University professor of special education Douglas Biklen, FC involves the use of a nondisabled "facilitator" to help a severely intellectually disabled and minimally or completely nonverbal "user" spell with a letterboard or keyboard through physical contact of some kind: supporting the user at the wrist, elbow, or shoulder, or even just holding the letterboard. The technique was immediately and enthusiastically embraced by the disability community, as individuals who had been deemed illiterate and profoundly cognitively impaired suddenly began proclaiming, as Peyton Goddard did the first time she was introduced to this technique, "I AM INTLGENT."[1]

Thousands of parents and professionals flocked to workshops hosted by the Facilitated Communication Institute (FCI), which Biklen established at Syracuse University in 1992, as well as other academic centers, including the University of Maine and the University of Wisconsin, to learn how to access this "unexpected literacy."[2] By the early 1990s, there were FC networks in thirty-eight states, and the practice was endorsed by both the Autism Society of America and The Association for the Severely Handicapped (TASH).[3] Psychologist Laura Schreibman has called the response to FC unprecedented: "There has been nothing in the history of autism treatment to rival the FC phenomenon."[4]

Particularly remarkable was how quickly FC was embraced in the absence of any research proving its validity. Biklen conducted no studies before introducing it to American audiences; his initial article celebrating the new intervention was published in the non-peer-reviewed, student-run *Harvard Educational Review*. Nevertheless, his claims were immediately picked up by the popular press, including the *New York Times*, *Time Magazine*, *Reader's Digest*, and the *Washington Post*, as well as by ABC's *Prime Time Live*.[5]

Biklen's report flew in the face of almost five decades of research—not only on autism, but across adjacent fields such as language and communication, infant behavior, and learning.[6] Many investigators considered his proposal "to redefine autism"[7]—from a cognitive impairment to "'motor' apraxia, a hypothesized disconnection between the motor and language systems of the brain that precludes direct communication"[8]—premature, particularly given the qualitative approach he had taken in his paper. But, as psychologist Gina Green recalls, "relatively few in developmental disabilities who knew how to test the claims about FC experimentally wanted to get involved," because "it was (is) not politically correct in many circles to suggest that FC might not be all it appears. . . . Those who do are likely to be labeled heretics, oppressors of the disabled, [and] inhumane."[9]

But a crisis quickly emerged that made the question of authorship increasingly urgent. In 1991, fourteen-year-old Jenny Storch, through FC, accused her father of raping her hundreds of times. And she wasn't the only one. By 1994 over five dozen cases of sexual abuse had been reported,[10] some resulting in the removal of children from their homes and the imprisonment of their parents.

These incidents catalyzed a thorough investigation into authorship in FC. The results were remarkably consistent. Across more than four dozen controlled experiments, users were only able to communicate information that was known to the facilitator. When the facilitator and user were given different information—the user was shown a picture of a shoe, for example, while the facilitator saw a key—any coherent output would reflect the facilitator's knowledge (i.e., the user would spell "key"). Emory psychologist Scott Lilienfeld summarized the early results, "In the 19 well-controlled studies of FC performed prior to 1999, the number of successful validations of FC was 0 out of 183."[11] Subsequent reviews in 2014 and 2018 found "unequivocal evidence for facilitator control: messages generated through FC are authored by the facilitators rather than the individuals with disabilities."[12] Not even a million-dollar prize offered by the James Randi Education Foundation could produce a validated demonstration of FC.[13] Ultimately, FC was rejected by every relevant professional organization, including the American Academy of Pediatrics, the American Association on Intellectual and Developmental Disabilities, the American Speech-Language-Hearing Association, and the American Psychological Association.

FC never completely disappeared—almost 90% of autism parents experiment with alternative treatments,[14] and it persisted alongside a host of other discredited interventions, such as diet, vitamins, brushing, and Auditory Integration Training, to name just a few. But its reputation was decidedly fringe. Syracuse University changed the name of the FCI to the Institute on Communication and Inclusion in 2010 to avoid the FC stigma, although they never disavowed the practice. And when Rutgers ethics professor Anna Stubblefield was convicted in 2015 of conducting a sexual relationship with a severely cognitively impaired man whose consent she procured through FC, the public fascination with the case—which received extensive coverage in the *New York Times Magazine*[15]—was motivated at least in part by the assumption that, as an academic, she should have known better.

So I was very surprised to hear, in 2019, that several parents from the Philadelphia area whom I had known for years were using a new iteration of FC, called Spell to Communicate (S2C), with their severely autistic sons. Created by Elizabeth Vosseller in 2013, S2C is very similar to the Rapid Prompting Method (RPM), which had been developed by Soma Mukhopadhyay for her severely autistic son Tito and brought to the United States a dozen years earlier. Unlike Biklen's style of FC, neither RPM nor S2C involve directly touching users—which is why proponents typically deny that the resulting production is facilitated.[16] But because both require another person to hold a letterboard while the user spells with an outstretched finger—and, critically, because users are typically unable to spell when the letterboard is fixed on a stand or table—researchers and clinicians outside the FC community classify RPM and S2C as FC variants that raise the same questions of authorship that have been central to this controversy since the 1990s. As psychologist James Todd explains, "You manipulate the output device or you manipulate the person, but that doesn't mean the output is valid."[17]

Like the previous chapters on guardianship and sheltered workshops, I had always intended to take an ethnographic approach to FC, so I was thrilled when the families I knew not only readily agreed to talk with me, but introduced me to a pair of practitioners who were teaching S2C out of an office half an hour from my house.

I was very clear from the beginning that my research had left me skeptical, but that it was important to me to accurately and thoroughly represent my subjects' experience with S2C. And at first they seemed enthusiastic. I conducted about a dozen hours of interviews in 2020, including one with an S2C user who spelled out his answers to my questions on a letterboard held by his mother. But then something changed. First one, then another, then a third of my interlocutors withdrew their permission for me to use our conversations in my book.

A journalist friend told me that it was too late to revoke consent. But I was less concerned about legality than I was about leaving my interlocutors feeling disrespected or betrayed. So I turned instead to the same type of source material on which I based my historical analysis. There is an extensive archive of memoirs about FC, written by parents as well as by users—including three published while I was working on this book. Like the narratives discussed earlier, these all celebrate the liberation of intact minds from their autistic prisons. At the same time, the reports of these committed FC proponents inadvertently raise the same concerns about agency that critics have cited for the past three decades, ultimately foregrounding the question that motivated this entire project: Are there tangible harms that follow the assumption of the intact mind?

* * *

FC memoirs look very much like other intact mind memoirs at the outset. The children are similarly described as profoundly impaired. At nine years old, Portia Iversen's son Dov is "not able to speak, or to communicate in any way, or play with toys, or be left alone for a few moments without endangering himself."[18] Dianne Goddard cites from a report detailing her daughter Peyton's behavior at the age of twenty-two, just before her introduction to FC: "Violent incidents of hitting at school and home. . . . Attempting to eat items on floor or outside: dirt, sticks, trash. . . . She cannot be left alone, nor is she capable of being in public places."[19] And J. B. Handley's son Jamie is considered illiterate and innumerate, governed by compulsions such as shredding leaves, and prone to fierce episodes of self-injury that have "sent him to the emergency room."[20]

Despite these significant disabilities, the authors routinely use the same intact mind imagery that has defined autism parent memoirs since *The Siege*. Valerie Gilpeer notes that, before FC, her daughter Emily seemed "as if she were locked inside herself. . . . She appeared to live in an isolated space to which we had repeatedly tried to gain access and failed. She was alone in there."[21] Matthew and Nancy Hobson straightforwardly titled their memoir, *I'm So Glad You Found Me in Here*;[22] Peyton Goddard's early years were defined by her mother's struggle to "prove that [psychological] evaluations do not reflect [Peyton's] abilities . . . I know my baby girl is smart."[23] This faith and effort is rewarded when those intact minds are discovered through FC, in dramatic transformations that parallel those in non-FC narratives.

However, there is a notable difference: in non-FC memoirs, typical cognition is just part of an *overall* normalization. In other words, at the end of these books the children and young adults are virtually indistinguishable from neurotypical peers: fully verbal, social, independent, and devoid of the most disruptive symptoms that often accompany the disorder, such as self-injury, perseveration, rigidity, and self-stimulatory behaviors like hand-flapping or spinning. Susan Levin reports that her son Ben "seems to have let go of most of the autistic behaviors (e.g., nonresponsiveness, checking out, lack of interest or motivation, lack of energy, etc.)."[24] And, in one of the many passages he contributed to the coauthored account *There's a Boy in Here*, Sean Barron describes how he discovered that he was "*separate from the problems I had and that I could overcome them. I declared war! I was going to fight against all the behaviors I had obeyed all my life*" (emphasis in original).[25] Several have officially lost their diagnosis. Both Patricia Stacey and Jenny McCarthy describe encounters with professionals who pronounce, as Stacey's provider does, " 'We do not believe your son has autism' ";[26] an evaluator from the state department similarly marvels at McCarthy's son Evan, " 'This isn't autism anymore. . . . We have never seen a recovery like this.' "[27]

In contrast, even after the intact mind has been accessed, the subjects of FC memoirs are still profoundly impaired, requiring round-the-clock supervision and assistance with the most basic activities of daily living. And challenging behavior often remains a significant problem. Although DJ Savarese had "completely caught up with his [sixth grade] peers, even surpassed them in some respects," he still "hit his aides and resource room teacher and acted out in a number of classes."[28] Elizabeth Bonker's mother Virginia Breen reports in an epilogue to their memoir, "Almost every day [for the past eighteen months], all day, someone has to sit beside [Elizabeth] to deflect her fists or knees from hitting her face."[29] Peyton Goddard, who in 2002 became the first FC user to graduate as valedictorian from an American college, disrupted classes with periodic meltdowns—such as one in her Intermediate Algebra class, which her mother describes: "Suddenly, with no warning, Peyton stands up and begins yelling a prolonged, primordial cry. She screams while overturning the table."[30] As Russell Martin reflects about his nephew Ian, "his parents and sister, like everyone who was close to him, of course had hoped—had secretly been certain—that this remarkable new means of expressing himself would tend to quiet his all-too-regular distress, and now it seemed plainly probable that that never would be the case."[31]

To explain the enormous gap between their children's behavior and their facilitated articulation, insight, and academic achievement, these parent authors offer Biklen's "motor apraxia" theory—which, as Martin paraphrases, reframes autism as a disorder "in which people with normal and sometimes even sophisticated intellects, as well as commensurate linguistic abilities, are trapped inside bodies they can't control."[32] Ralph Savarese uses similar imagery to describe the "intact mind trapped inside of [his son DJ's] uncooperative body."[33] And FC users themselves explain their lived experience with severe autism the same way. Naoki Higashida, who spelled the bestselling *The Reason I Jump* with facilitation, reports that autistic individuals "don't even have proper control over our own bodies . . . it's as if we're remote-controlling a faulty robot."[34] Echoes Emily Grodin, who cowrote a memoir with her mother, "*Lots of us are trapped inside bodies not connected to our mind*" (emphasis in original).[35]

It's a scary image, one that evokes locked-in syndrome, the condition in which a patient is completely paralyzed but fully conscious—most famously described in the 1997 memoir *The Diving Bell and the Butterfly*, which Jean-Dominique Bauby dictated solely by blinking his left eye, the only voluntary movement of which he was capable. However, as frequently as the motor or global apraxia theory of autism has been promoted by the FC community, it has found little traction outside of it. Speech-language pathologist Diane Twachtman-Cullen sums up the literature: "The unidimensional view of autism as essentially a movement disorder stands in stark contrast to research findings."[36]

About a quarter of autistic kids do suffer from childhood apraxia of speech (CAS), a "speech sound disorder in which the precision and consistency of the articulatory movements of speech are impaired in the absence of . . . neuromuscular deficits."[37] But the motor problems caused by CAS are extremely localized. Nowhere, outside of FC papers, is there any evidence that autistic children exhibit a global or pervasive apraxia that would so greatly impair their overall movement. As speech pathologist Howard Shane points out, the opposite is often true, noting that "exemplary motor skills are frequently associated with this disability."[38] And the memoirs bear this out: Emily Grodin participates in dance class and soccer;[39] Jamie Handley rides an adult tricycle;[40] Peyton Goddard skis and swims;[41] Ido Kedar loves his scooter.[42] Fine motor control is also evidenced, as the subjects of FC memoirs are described assembling 300-piece puzzles,[43] eating with silverware,[44] and playing piano[45] without any physical support whatsoever. Kedar even acknowledges that these inconsistencies defy explanation: "It is so strange that I can't do what I want. . . . I really don't understand why my body can listen to my thoughts some of the time and other times my body refuses to listen."[46]

Not only do individuals with autism not typically evidence global motor difficulties, but on the flip side, patients who do have significant movement disturbances—such as cerebral palsy (CP) or Parkinson's disease—can virtually always communicate independently,[47] even if all they can do is blink their eyes or blow into a straw. In her memoir about her nonverbal son with severe CP, for example, Marianne Leone recounts how a communication system was built around "Jesse's only volitional movement, a raking grasp. We installed a program . . . that scanned through the alphabet one letter at a time, speaking it aloud. To choose the letter he wanted, Jesse would pull on a little green alien connected to a switch on the computer." Note that this method required absolutely no physical support from another person.[48]

Ultimately, the motor apraxia theory of autism dissolves into a tautology, in which evidence derived solely from observing FC is then used to legitimate it, as psychologists John Jacobson, James Mulick, and Allen Schwartz explain: "It is inferred that because this literacy [exhibited through FC] implies intellectual ability in the normal-to-superior range, these nonverbal children and adults must have motor disorders that prevent the expression of competence vocally, manually, or gesturally."[49]

If the motor apraxia theory has little evidence behind it, there is on the other hand robust support for Michael Rutter's 1968 claim that "the language disorder in autism is the primary abnormality." What is so compelling about his review of the research more than fifty years ago is how neatly the findings from a range of studies by different investigators converged. For example, autistic children performed poorly on assessments requiring "verbal concepts, abstraction, or symbolization . . . even on *tests which do not require [them] to speak* (such as a test which requires [them] to place a series of pictures in an order which conveys a story" (emphasis in original). This is exactly what would be expected from a more pervasive language impairment, as opposed to a problem of simply articulating speech sounds.[50]

Rutter also summarizes experiments by psychologists Neil O'Connor and Beate Hermelin comparing the abilities of neurotypical, intellectually disabled, and autistic children to memorize strings of words. They found that neurotypical and intellectually disabled subjects attended to the meaning of words—they would group words they had been asked to remember by categories, such as colors or numbers, and they could memorize longer strings of words if they were assembled into coherent units rather than just randomly arranged. In contrast, as Rutter reports, "the verbal recall of autistic children was relatively independent of the *meaning* of what they had heard. These results tend to suggest a hypothesis in terms of deficits in verbal coding and patterning" (emphasis in original).[51]

Importantly, language deficits persist even in autistic individuals who can talk. One of the reasons Lorna Wing introduced the autism "spectrum" more than a decade after the publication of Rutter's paper was that even the most mildly affected individuals diagnosed with Asperger's syndrome exhibited, along with the problems with social interaction and repetitive behavior displayed by Kanner's more disabled patients, significant impairments in communication. Although the ability to speak is unaffected, Wing noted, "the content of speech is impoverished."[52] Subsequent research has delineated the many forms this impoverishment may take: difficulty understanding metaphors and inferences,[53] as well as humor and irony;[54] trouble comprehending words and concepts describing emotional[55] or mental[56] states; failure to provide context, respond appropriately, avoid non sequiturs, and otherwise maintain conversational reciprocity.[57] These factors have led one team of researchers to hypothesize that "autism may be a generalized disorder of complex information processing."[58]

As I worked through this literature, I couldn't help thinking about my friend's autistic son, Max, who is so obsessed with ceiling fans that he once texted me, pretending to be his father, to set up a time for the family to visit so he could check out our one ceiling fan. Whenever I see him, the first five minutes of our conversation is always the same: Why do I have so few ceiling fans? Where is it in my house? What brand? Do I think I will ever get more?

Max is much less disabled than the autistic subjects of FC memoirs: he is a fully verbal college graduate who will doubtlessly live independently one day. Yet it is his communication that reflects the perseveration, rigidity, and lack of social awareness that has been known to characterize autistic speech for decades, while the products of FC notably do not. Nor do they exhibit oddities such as pronoun reversal, incorrect verb tenses, or echolalia (the tendency to repeat fragments heard elsewhere) that are common not only in more severe manifestations of autism in general, but often in the speech patterns of FC users themselves.

Instead, the output generated through FC is notably abstract and sophisticated, both in syntax and content—which even the neurotypical authors sometimes have difficulty reconciling with the minimal education the users had received in special education classrooms. Russell Martin admits, "I couldn't help but wonder how [his nephew Ian] had come by this budding poetic sensibility."[59] Nancy Hobson similarly reflects, "It just didn't seem possible that [Matthew] had been able to absorb so much knowledge on his own . . . [but when his brother asked] 'How many world championships has Michael Jordan won?' Matthew knew the answer. He also knew about Desert Storm and the war in Kuwait."[60]

Ralph Savarese explores this gap in the greatest depth:

> Through typing, DJ is able to answer questions like "What is a mummy?" or "What is a capital?" He also knew about rich and poor passengers on the Titanic. . . .
>
> How to account for a neurologically disabled fourth-grader with both class and existential consciousness? How did DJ know these things? How, with almost no training in math, could he do complicated addition, subtraction, multiplication, and division problems in his head? How? . . . Later, when I'd start investigating this phenomenon, I'd discover that nobody really had an adequate theory

> beyond a notion of the child with autism somehow storing information (without exactly understanding it) and accessing it once he or she had come to communicative life.[61]

How? J. B. Handley actually asks his son this question, in a Q&A section of their coauthored memoir: "How were you able to teach yourself to read, spell, and do math?"—which, despite his father's admission that, "If you'd asked me back then [before S2C] if I thought Jamie could add, I would have said 'no,'" very quickly extended to calculus. And Jamie answers, "I think how I did it will remain unknown because I have no idea."[62]

Researchers, however, do have an idea. The consensus, in the mainstream psychological literature, is that the products of FC are not generated by the users but by the facilitators, who unconsciously direct the interaction through a host of involuntary movements known as ideomotor effects. First identified by William Carpenter in 1852 and popularized by William James almost forty years later, these effects also explain a range of phenomena including Ouija boards, divining rods, table turning, and automatic writing.[63]

Perhaps the most famous example of ideomotor effects is Clever Hans, the horse who captivated the citizens of Berlin in 1904 with his amazing abilities to answer questions about music, math, and other subjects by tapping his right hoof and moving his nose. A commission of experts—including two zoo directors, a veterinarian, two academics, and a circus manager—concluded after a full examination "that this was done without trickery on the part of human beings." It wasn't until a graduate student in psychology, Oskar Pfungst, undertook a series of controlled experiments with Hans that it was discovered that the horse was responding to extraordinarily subtle visual cues (such as very slightly bowing the head) that his interrogators likely had no idea they were exhibiting. At the same time, magazines across the Atlantic were reporting a similar American case: a dog named Roger who could not only do math, but translate words into French and German, purportedly by reading his owner's mind.[64]

This is not in any way to compare the intellectually and developmentally disabled to animals, but to illustrate that, while the most obvious concern about FC is manipulation through touch (that may occur as the facilitator adjusts the keyboard, modifies pressure on the hand, elbow, or shoulder, or simply shifts any part of the body that might brush against the user as they sit close together), how extensively—and virtually unnoticeably—behavior can be cued in the absence of any physical contact whatsoever.

Wolf Wolfensberger further suggests that perceived improvements in behavior or attention following the introduction of FC may be due to the

Hawthorne effect, named after research done at the Hawthorne Works of the Western Election Company almost a century ago "which showed that merely being paid attention could motivate people to greater performance."[65] For Howard Shane, the "influence that extensive and close human contact seems to have in reducing activity and increasing attention" is a provocative finding that might be incorporated into evidence-based interventions for this population.[66]

Beyond the factors actually shaping facilitated output, a host of cognitive traps may influence how these exchanges are interpreted. Social psychologist John V. Petrocelli suggests that FC believers are victims of the anecdotal fallacy, in which personal stories are used to justify broad truth claims. He also warns about the dangers of emotional reasoning, or "making misguided conclusions that something is true because one 'feels' it strongly while ignoring or discounting evidence to the contrary."[67] William Paul Simmons, Janyce Boynton, and Todd Landman point out the role of confirmation bias, in which we not only seek out evidence that supports what we already believe, but reject all disconfirming information.[68] Particularly striking in these memoirs—most of them written years or sometimes decades after the flood of controlled studies locating authorship with facilitators—is how little they engage with this literature. All Nancy Hobson says in the 2010 account she coauthored with her son is that "researchers could not explain how FC worked, so their doubts and skepticism grew."[69] Even in 2021, J. B. Handley "didn't know or care much about this whole controversy."[70]

But proponents have never addressed any of these well-established psychological phenomena in their defense of FC, which rests instead on several problematic assertions. The first "proof," as Biklen labeled it in his *Harvard Educational Review* paper, is that "some students were able to type independently."[71] Almost thirty years later, Ralph Savarese argues that "independent typ[ers] . . . d[o] away with the question of authorship altogether."[72] J. B. Handley agrees, citing spellers who start with support but end up "typ[ing] independently" as "all you need to disprove ASHA [the American Speech-Language-Hearing Association, which has issued a position statement rejecting all forms of FC], you just need to hear from them."[73]

The thorny question, of course, is what exactly is meant by "independence"? Biklen classified users as independent as long as their hands were not being directly supported, even if they required touch "on the shoulder, leg, thread of the sleeve, or other location" in order to communicate.[74] Contemporary debates over FC rely on a much more intuitive definition of independence, pointing to prominent users whose videos show them spelling on fixed keyboards with no person touching them in any way.

But these celebrities' accomplishments unfold amid a troubling context: they may not require direct touch to communicate, but they typically cannot spell without the presence of a certain person or persons. Ido Kedar reports that, although he still prefers to spell with a letterboard, he has progressed to typing on a fixed keyboard. But he still "need[s] a person nearby to help me keep my focus," he explains. "Or I return so easily to my internal world which makes no demands and provides a drug-like trance to boot."[75]

Portia Iversen includes a similar example of this phenomenon in *Strange Son*, which recounts how she brought Soma Mukhopadhyay, the founder of RPM, and her son Tito—arguably the world's most famous speller and now the author of eight books—to the United States from India. Tito spells on a letterboard and writes on a legal pad with no physical assistance. But one day, Iversen tries to engage with Tito when his mother isn't present:

> I tried to make contact with Tito on my own. . . . I held the alphabet board in front of him, just as I'd seen Soma do. "Tito, how are you today?" I asked, tapping on the alphabet board. Nothing. It felt as if I were asking a tree. . . . I continued, trying desperately to make the most rudimentary connection with the being who stood unresponsively before me. . . . Why couldn't Tito communicate with anyone but Soma?[76]

Later in the book, Iversen recounts how Soma and Tito agreed to be tested by neuroscientists at the University of California, San Francisco, but when the researchers read Tito a story with Soma out of the room, he was unable to answer a single question about it. Somewhat surprisingly, these episodes evoke no doubt in Iversen. Although she sees Soma "urge Tito on, with abrupt verbal prompts and sweeping gestures [from across the room]," she's convinced "there was no way [Soma] could have signaled Tito to produce . . . complex, unpredictable, naturalistic conversation."[77] No doubt, this is exactly why, throughout history, luminaries like Sir Arthur Conan Doyle[78] and University of Pennsylvania professor of chemistry Robert Hare[79] have embraced Ouija boards, table turning, and other examples of ideomotor effects. It's just so hard to believe that barely or completely imperceptible movements could possibly have such consequential impact.

Another type of evidence cited repeatedly in FC memoirs as sufficient and definitive proof of validity is the communication of information by users that is unknown to facilitators. Some examples are surprisingly vague, such as J. B. Handley's curt dismissal of the possibility of influence, "I will just share this simple fact: Jamie spelled things with [his facilitator] that she didn't know. Enough said."[80]

Others are more specific. Russell Martin recounts how, a week after he started typing with FC, "Claudia [Ian's mother], who hadn't yet heard what they'd encountered, typed TODAY DAD AND I SAW A, before bringing Ian's hand to the keyboard, steadying it, pulling it firmly back following each sharp keystroke that soon spelled COYOYE. It was the first time Claudia had not known what the appropriate final word would be, her initial proof to herself that she was not subconsciously willing the proper keystrokes."[81]

This story certainly has potential to validate the authenticity of Ian's communication, but it also raises important questions. Howard Shane advises, "Avoid basing judgement about FC success on labeling tasks alone, because naming (and spelling) the labels of common objects is frequently a skill that marginal spellers possess."[82] In other words, a key piece of information required to assess the validity of particular facilitated exchanges—but one that is often not disclosed by proponents—is the level of literacy exhibited without facilitation. It turns out that, before he was ever introduced to FC, Ian was performing above grade level academically, with a "reading vocabulary also above the first-grade level," so it seems likely he could produce a word resembling "coyote" on his own. That doesn't mean we shouldn't question whether he could author an insightful assessment of his own disorder: "I NBNEVER RWEALLY LIKED COWWS THAT MUCH. IJUST NEEDED RTHEM FOR MTY ROUTINE."[83]

Another example of validation in the natural environment raises different concerns. Jennifer Binder Le-Pape—one of the members of my local S2C group, actually—published an essay on the website of the S2C organization I-ASC (International Association for Spelling as Communication) in which she describes how her son Alex "is capable of communicating information that is unknown to us but can be verified by a neutral third party":

> One morning he went and got his letterboard and handed it to me. When I asked him what was up, he spelled "I need to go to the doctor." I asked him why and he replied "Ears hurt, throat hurts." There was no external evidence of this—no fever, his appetite had seemed normal at breakfast, he wasn't pulling at or holding his ear. We went to have him checked out by the doctor, who confirmed that one ear was indeed infected, the other had a significant amount of fluid pressing on the inner ear, and his throat was irritated by post-nasal drip. So to summarize, **Alex told me something I could not have otherwise known, which was then confirmed by a professional with absolutely no stake one way or another in how he communicates**[84] (emphasis in original).

This is another provocative example. But it's impossible to rule out other ways LePape might have known her son was sick—Clever Hans is nothing if not a cautionary tale about how easy it is to send and receive signals without knowing it. As Alex's mother, LePape is no doubt very sensitive to his emotions and behavior, and may have inferred from very minor departures from baseline that he wasn't feeling well. As researchers have pointed out, there are many possible explanations behind reports of information communicated through FC that was not known by facilitators. Facilitators may not remember previously being exposed to such details—either through past encounters, access to client records, or casually chatting with parents. They may know their clients well enough to make informed guesses in response to questions about their activities or preferences. Or unorthodox spelling in FC output might invite subjective interpretation by facilitators.[85]

As complicated as it is to tease out facilitator influence in uncontrolled settings, it is actually very easy to test in the lab. Investigators primarily rely on one of two strategies: a "message passing" test, in which users are asked to communicate information which the facilitator does not know, or a "double blind" paradigm, in which the user and facilitator are given either the same or different information, which the user is then asked to relay back to the researcher. In a review of controlled studies reported in 17 journals and 8 conference papers including over 200 subjects, Gina Green concluded, "Many messages were produced over numerous trials and sessions, but the vast majority were accurate and appropriate to context only when the facilitator knew what was to be produced."[86]

I'm not saying that every single message ever produced through FC originated with the facilitator. If there's one thing I truly believe, after two decades of living in the world of severe autism, it's that the mind and all its potential anomalies—from the savants who multiply five-digit numbers in their heads to the baby born without 80% of his brain who somehow survived for five years—represents an unfathomable mystery. But what I am saying is that—given everything we know about language development, ideomotor effects, and facilitator influence; given the consequential decisions that have been made through FC about guardianship, medication, sexual activity, education, residence, and other central concerns; given that even some of the most committed pro-FC researchers have described the intervention as "fragile vis-à-vis its reliability"[87]—perhaps the most incomprehensible thing about the entire debate is that proponents so firmly reject controlled testing.

Douglas Biklen took this stance in his first paper on FC, advising prospective facilitators, "Don't use teaching or communication situations to 'test' the person."[88] Why not? Testing was too confrontational and anxiety-producing, he would later elaborate: "Failure on authorship tests of facilitated communication could leave testees classified as severely or profoundly retarded. . . .

Who but they are to say what amount of terror, confusion, and defeat they may feel upon entering, enduring, or exiting the test?"[89] Soma Mukhopadhyay, the founder of RPM, similarly claims on her website, "I am against any research where students are put in stressful or testing situations—having to prove their intelligence is insulting and demeaning."[90]

Anxiety features heavily in proponents' explanations of why users fail controlled tests, but it's not the only reason. Also blamed are "word-finding problems" autistic people allegedly suffer from that prevent them from making correct identifications,[91] as well as short-term memory issues that keep them from recounting recent events. FC user Gregory Tino defends the latter theory in his memoir: "Critics of the letterboard view [the inability to answer questions] as evidence that we are being influenced by our communication partner who doesn't know the memory being asked of us. It is not true. It is that we have memory retrieval problems!"[92]

The issue is not whether autistic individuals are prone to anxiety (up to 70% of those on the spectrum do meet the diagnostic criteria for at least one psychiatric comorbidity[93]) or whether they have word retrieval or memory problems (of this there's no evidence). But if any of these factors really interfered with users' ability to participate in the testing process, then, as Gina Green points out, they "should have been manifested when facilitators both did and did not know the expected answers. Instead, correct words were 'found' on most trials when the facilitator was given corresponding information, very few when they were not."[94] Facilitator influence has proven to be such a persistent and vexing problem in controlled tests that Anne Donnellan, director of the Autism Program at the University of San Diego, and her colleague Paul Haskew tried to moot the entire controversy by claiming that autistic children spelled what their facilitators saw instead of what they themselves were shown because they were psychic.[95]

Rather than flat-out rejecting lab-based tests, as proponents of RPM and earlier forms of FC have done, the S2C community has taken a different tack. While practitioners and families similarly refuse the simple, controlled experiments that have historically been used to reveal facilitator influence (Jennifer Binder LePape opens her blog post with the declaration, "Let me cut right to the chase: no, [her son Alex] won't do a message passing test for you"[96]), sympathetic investigators have claimed to prove, or are currently trying to prove, authorship through increasingly advanced technologies, including eye tracking devices,[97] functional magnetic resonance imaging (fMRI),[98] and accelerometry.[99] But these attempts to bedazzle a public that associates fancy tech with cutting-edge science still can't credibly explain how researchers have consistently demonstrated facilitator influence with nothing more sophisticated than some pictures and manila folders.

* * *

When I was doing the interviews that I thought would be the basis for this chapter, I thought about taking Jonah to the S2C practitioners near me. I had always assumed that he wouldn't be a candidate, because he can type completely independently—nothing more advanced than the titles of the videos he wants to watch on YouTube, but his ability to accurately tap the letters on his iPad (and before that, on an iPod) with his stubby fingers, permanently swollen from years of pounding on tables and walls, surely precluded the motor impairments that allegedly necessitate the use of FC. Perhaps the most unanticipated finding I discovered during my research was that many FC users actually share Jonah's basic literacy, and his abilities to both speak and type words or short phrases. Elizabeth Bonker, writes her mother Virginia Breen, says " 'pizza' . . . when she sees a sign for her favorite food. . . . 'Fire' is another favorite word, which she says when we light birthday candles or burn wood in the fireplace."[100] And Gregory Tino reports, via FC, "I can recite almost everything from a movie or TV show, but I can't hold a conversation. Why is that? It seems to be easier for me to say scripted things instead of thoughts that I make up myself." Why it should be easier, or the nature of the brain impairment that would preclude someone with typical language capabilities from independently typing complete, complex sentences but allow him to, as Tino does, search for favorite commercials on YouTube without support, is never satisfactorily explained.[101]

I have to admit, I was curious: Would Jonah sit for a lesson? Would I be able to see the board shift, or hear a change in the instructor's pitch, or observe any movements of her body that might serve as unintentional cues?

And yes, of course I wondered what he would spell. After all the studies I'd read, I didn't really believe it would be him, so I can't explain why I found the prospect so tantalizing. Maybe I just wanted to pretend, for an hour, that Jonah could understand the expansive universe beyond home, his day program, and Costco. That everything that is meaningful to me—from history to literature to philosophy to politics—would be meaningful to him, that I could ask, "What do you think?" and he could answer. Maybe I just wanted to break open the tightly scripted exchanges that structure our days, where Jonah says, "People, sisters, and all animals, I'll be right back," and I say, "People, sisters, and all animals, one more time," or he says, "Waterpark WITH Jen," and I say, "When you see Jen [who might be a bubbly Villanova student who worked with Jonah fifteen years ago, or might be someone I don't remember from the various programs he's attended since then], you should definitely ask her." Maybe I just wanted him to surprise me.

When I told my husband about my plan, he simply asked, "And what will you do if he accuses you of abuse?"

It was a reminder of what I already knew: FC is not a parlor game or a research project, but a "pseudoscience"[102] or even a "pathological science"[103] that poses multiple and significant risks to an extraordinarily vulnerable population. The worst harm isn't the false abuse allegations that have resulted in users being removed from their families, or even the very real abuse that has been justified by FC—such as the case of Australian facilitator Martina Susanne Schweiger who, similar to Anna Stubblefield, was convicted in 2014 of engaging in a sexual relationship with a severely autistic client whose consent was solicited through FC;[104] or the even more tragic case of Gigi Jordan, who killed her eight-year-old son in 2010 after, she claims, he told her through FC that he wanted to commit suicide to escape the abuse of his father and stepfather (which has never been documented).[105] Fortunately, these outcomes are not common.

Nor is the worst harm the expense—although it is tremendous, in both dollars and time. A very recent 2022 study calculated that RPM in particular costs school districts $32,159 per student to implement the first year alone, and almost $28,000/year in ongoing support "with little evidence of positive outcomes."[106] Ido Kedar's memoir nicely illustrates the opportunity cost: he describes how his parents dismissed his entire Applied Behavioral Analysis (ABA) team because the therapists evinced skepticism that it was actually Ido directing the output produced through RPM. He additionally scoffs at the Picture Exchange Communication System (PECS)—a popular, evidence-based intervention that allows nonverbal children to communicate by pointing to or handing over small pictures of what they want—because it "is not enough. It's so basic."[107]

No, the worst harm of all is that FC routinely hijacks the (albeit limited and very fragile) agency of profoundly disabled individuals. As psychologist Kathleen Dillon reports, "[FC] messages are often given more credibility than the utterances or behaviors of the subject,"[108] even though there is a robust literature supporting the communicative intent of both echolalic language and nonverbal behavior in autism.[109]

Examples arise again and again in these memoirs, as both the spoken words of the users and their actions are trumped by what is spelled on the letterboard. Ralph Savarese describes how, as he was trying to spell with his son, DJ "began to bang his head and signed, 'all done, all done.'" On another occasion, he tried to close the computer in the middle of a typing session.[110] But Savarese never even considers the obvious possibility that DJ finds interacting with the keyboard aversive. Naoki Higashida reveals that he doesn't really like playing with the toys he picks up, but would rather "get stuck in some difficult book or to debate some issue or other."[111] Ido Kedar notes that "I might really want to get a chicken dish for dinner in a restaurant, but if someone asks me if I want beef my mouth is often messing it up by saying 'yes.' "[112] And Russell Martin also recounts how, even as his nephew Ian typed that he wanted to go to school, "he kept kicking and screaming, 'Stay home! Sick! Stay home!" Instead of interpreting both his words and behavior as clear evidence he did not want to go to school, Ian's parents decided that his "outward behavior, his apparent contentment or pleasure as well as his rage, was not evidence they could depend on":

> Always his family had assumed that he found great security and reassurance in watching [his favorite movies] time after time after time. But what he wanted, he now was saying instead, was *please* to see some new stuff. The movies he had watched every day for six months, some for a year or more, had long since become DREAFFULLY VBORING. . . . Yet with each acquiescence, each obviously empathetic attempt on his parents' part to comply with his request [to read a new book, or try honey], Ian responded by screaming, by fighting the new experience as if it were likely to be lethal, his typed words always antithetical to his physical reactions. . . . Repeatedly now, Claudia and Boyce pressed the question: Should we believe what you say or what you type? And his response, like this one, always was unequivocal: YOI SHOULD DO WHATT I TYPE. . . . But each attempt to introduce him to new foods, new activities, new books and movies at unusual times of the day, was met with nothing less than a kind of physical terror at the prospect of the impending change.[113]

Gregory Tino adds, "I may say 'yes' when I mean 'no' and vice versa. . . . My mom has learned to always ask me on the letterboard instead of verbally. The only way to get my true answer is for me to spell it out. . . . By my vocalizations and actions, you might think that I love Barney . . . but I actually hate him!"[114]

As the mother of a twenty-four-year-old autistic son who still watches *Sesame Street* constantly, this gets me, every time.

Not so Neurodiversity advocates. In a profound and frankly incomprehensible irony, the same organizations that fight so hard to limit or even eliminate guardianship because of the restrictions it imposes on autonomy—such as the Autistic Self-Advocacy Network, the Arc, and the National Disability

Rights Network—also signed a letter to the board of directors of the American Speech-Language-Hearing Association in 2018 urging the withdrawal of the organization's position statements against FC.[115] And their support of these interventions remains unqualified, despite the obvious undermining of autonomy represented by the thousands of examples of facilitator influence documented in the literature, each one representing another cognitively impaired person literally turned into a puppet.

Ultimately, it's this "unwitting ventriloquism" that marks FC not only as bad practice, but as, more fundamentally, "an abuse of human rights."[116] Multiple scholars have argued that FC violates several articles in the 2006 United Nations Convention on the Rights of Persons with Disabilities discussed in the previous chapter—including Article 12, which protects the disabled from "undue influence"; Article 16, which "prevent[s] all forms of exploitation"; Article 17, which preserves "physical and mental integrity"; and Article 21, which defends "freedom of expression."[117] Similar rights-based justifications anchor the position statements of several professional organizations, such as ASHA and the International Society for Augmentative and Alternative Communication.

And yet, despite these human rights concerns, despite the overwhelming scientific consensus, FC is enjoying what one 2018 paper has described as a "resurgence." Up to 10% of autistic children in some regions of the country have tried it;[118] a 2019 study found that RPM was more frequently used by the teachers they surveyed than evidence-based practices like PECS or video modeling.[119] In fact, I had to keep revising this chapter, as facilitated individuals were repeatedly celebrated in the news for extraordinary accomplishments. In May 2022, spellers David Teplitz and Hari Srinivasen graduated from the University of California at Berkeley; Srinivasen—well known to the autism community since his appointment to the Interagency Autism Coordinating Committee (IACC), which advises NIH on how to spend its autism research dollars—will next pursue a fully funded doctorate in neuroscience at Vanderbilt. The same month, Elizabeth Bonker was named the valedictorian of Rollins College, more than eleven years after the publication of her memoir. In her pre-recorded address, delivered via text-to-speech software with the press of a button, Bonker vowed to expand typing access to the "31 million nonspeakers with autism in the world" and break them out of their "silent cage."[120]

What was particularly striking about these stories—which were reported by many prominent news platforms, including NPR, CNN, *USA Today*, *Newsweek*, and others—was their uniformly uncritical tone. Even though one journalist reported that David Teplitz "taps one letter at a time . . . without looking at the keyboard"—something that even expert touch-typists can't do without input from all ten fingers to orient their hands[121]—she failed to consult with a single source that might have pointed her to the extensive literature debunking FC.[122] Researcher Gina Green's 1994 assessment that FC skeptics are "likely to be labeled heretics, oppressors of the disabled, [and] inhumane," quoted at the beginning of this chapter, has never seemed more prescient.

With autism incidence skyrocketing to 1 in 44 American children affected, and almost half a million intellectually and developmentally disabled individuals waiting for services, we have never needed evidence-based treatments more. As desperate parents turn to increasingly risky interventions such as chemical castration, stem cell therapy, and bleach enemas, James Todd argues for a "moral obligation to be empirical . . . to protect everyone from the trap of our own biases and distorted thinking."[123]

Instead, the opposite is occurring. And this is where FC memoirs converge with many of the other intact mind narratives discussed in Chapters 2 and 3: personal experience trumps science, whose orthodox representatives are dismissed as useless, self-interested reactionaries, too invested in their limited strategies to recognize the miracle unfolding right under their noses. J. B. Handley congratulates S2C founder Elizabeth Vosseller for "throwing seventy years of autism research out the window and saying every expert in the field is wrong."[124] Agrees Ido Kedar, "I know [Soma Mukhopadhyay, the creator of RPM] is doubted by the experts. But maybe they are experts with books and diplomas, not insight. Soma is insightful. She gives non-verbal autistic kids hope. That's a blessing because too often my experts brought me only desperation."[125]

I get hope. Hope is a lifeline to the completely ordinary future all parents want for their kids. A life of virtually limitless options—from the big decisions, like where to live or work, to the seemingly insignificant inclinations to order a pizza or even just open the door and take a walk. Accepting a child's complete and lifelong dependence can be paralyzing. As Virginia Breen reflects, "In Dante's *Inferno*, above the gates of hell a sign reads, 'Abandon all hope.' I cannot think of a more apt description of hell—a place without hope. Yet the burden of autism can push us to live in that very place. . . . Somehow, autism moms have to find a way to cling to hope with a tenacity that is stronger than autism's grip on our children. But how?"[126]

For these parents, it's by seizing on any evidence of their children's intact minds. Facilitated IQ tests and the genius scores they inevitably reveal replace the loss of diagnosis that features so prominently in many non-FC intact mind narratives. When Ido Kedar is permitted to use his letterboard during a neuropsychological evaluation, recounts his mother Tracy, "he soared from a low intellectual functioning score to that of an extremely bright child. . . . At the age of ten it was determined that he had a twelfth grade vocabulary."[127] Elizabeth Bonker's IQ soared from 69 at first test to 164 with facilitation.[128]

Even when specific test results aren't shared, the relief at establishing competency is palpable. Nothing is worse, in these memoirs, than intellectual disability. Dianne Goddard shudders, "Even long before I was a mother, a diagnosis of mental retardation seemed to me a fate worse than any incurable disease for a child . . . *retarded*. The word pained me more than any other, including, even, *death*."[129] Ralph Savarese directs readers to "Imagine . . . sending nonspeaking people with autism back to the mines of special ed, with labels of mental retardation."[130] Gregory Tino states, "It is infuriating to me when people call us retarded! It is one of the most hurtful things that you can say to me."[131] Hurtful, and, it is implied, inaccurate—not just for Tino, but for all those included under the umbrella of "us." Which might be everyone ever diagnosed with autism. J. B. Handley recounts a question he posed to S2C founder Elizabeth Vosseller: " 'Of all the nonspeaking kids who have come through your doors to seek therapy, how many have truly had a cognitive disability?' Her answer? 'None so far.' . . . These nonspeakers all over the world with an autism label, they are all like Jamie. . . . They are all brilliant people."[132]

Talk about a high-octane hope, one capable of physically and spiritually strengthening parents engaged every day in the extraordinarily difficult care of teen and even adult children who can't, despite the formidable intellects revealed through FC, ever be left alone.[133] "Loving someone is easy when you feel them loving you back," Virginia Breen gently chides her readers. "What happens when you feel that you are pouring your love into a black hole where no light shines out?"[134] David Mitchell, the translator of *The Reason I Jump*, further elucidates this almost material dimension of hope in his introduction. Naoki Higashida's facilitated narrative, Mitchell reveals, restored his belief in the typical capacity of his own autistic son and motivated him to work harder: "When you know that your kid wants to speak with you, when you know that he's taking in his surroundings every bit as attentively as your nonautistic daughter, whatever the evidence to the contrary, then you can be ten times more patient, willing, understanding and communicative; and ten times better able to help his development."[135]

Whatever the evidence to the contrary. Putting aside all the controlled studies and expert theories about the core deficits of autism, the authors of FC memoirs include so much evidence to the contrary, I constantly wondered why their editors didn't intervene. As discussed earlier, these include failed validation tests, ongoing aggressive and self-injurious behaviors, and instances when FC users contradicted, in their own rudimentary, spoken language, what they spelled on their letterboards.

But nowhere is the incredible contortion required to preserve the belief in the intact mind more apparent than in those instances, and there are several, where parents try to explain why their children consistently refuse to spell with them, but will do so with paid facilitators. Logically, this is one of the hardest inconsistencies to reconcile in the FC debate: that anyone, after a lifetime of alleged imprisonment in an intransigent body, would refuse to utilize her newly mastered communication strategy with her closest caregivers—those who not only love her most, but more practically, fulfill her daily needs. Recounts Valerie Gilpeer, "We [she and her husband Tom] tried with Emily again and again, but her ability to type with me and Tom didn't change. She typed with her psychologist, with Darlene, with other FC practitioners, with Anna and other autistic people. Just not with us."[136] Portia Iversen, struggling to spell with Dov, reflects longingly, "Soma had become almost like a clairvoyant, leading séances in her little booth where the children would learn and communicate as they could with no one else."[137] Explains Ido Kedar, who will spell with his mother but not his father, "It's weird because I can love someone and enjoy their company and know they believe in me and still resist pointing with them."[138]

I keep picturing Valerie and Emily, sitting in silence, waiting for a facilitator to show up so Valerie can ask her daughter what she most wants to know, what all the parents of severely autistic kids want to know: *Why did you do that? What do you need? How can I help?* And I think that perhaps nothing is more indicative of the seductive power of the intact mind and what it signifies—the autonomy that precludes the need for guardianship, the opportunity for college and a meaningful career beyond the limits of a 14(c) program—than that parents would rather believe their children simply do not want to communicate with them than acknowledge the reality of the impaired mind.

Conclusion

Contemporary disability service provision is guided by the directive to "presume competence." Defined by speech-language pathologists Katie O'Neil and Rebecca McCarthy as "an approach that assumes the communicator has significant untapped cognitive-linguistic capacities,"[1] this command is really just another way of assuming the intact mind. It should come as no surprise that the phrase was first coined in 1990 by facilitated communication (FC) enthusiast Douglas Biklen,[2] although it quickly exploded beyond the small cohort of FC researchers and practitioners to become the mantra of the Neurodiversity Movement. Other lineages trace this idea back a bit farther, to a 1984 paper by a different FC proponent, Anne Donnellan—the same researcher who offered the telepathic abilities of autistic children as an explanation for FC—which proposed that educational programming be guided by "the least dangerous assumption," or the decision "which, if incorrect, will have the least dangerous effect on the student."[3] Presuming competence, it follows, is less dangerous than presuming incompetence.

But this mindset carries its own dangers, particularly as presumption has shaded for some proponents into an *insistence* on competence. Spell to Communicate (S2C) founder Elizabeth Vosseller claims success with literally 100% of the nonverbal children she sees;[4] so does Soma Mukhopadhyay, the creator of the Rapid Prompting Method (RPM).[5] Christopher Kliewer, Douglas Biklen, and Amy Petersen argue that intellectual disability is "no more objectively real than was the label *witch* imposed by male authorities onto some unfortunate women."[6]

It shades into the surreal, this ontological rejection of cognitive impairment as *not objectively real*. What to make, then, of Bill Davis's account of his son Chris's pica, a compulsion to eat inedible objects: "He was grinding his teeth into the plaster of the walls. He ate a hole in the drapes! He ate his clothing. He ate ants, nails, mud"?[7] Or Robert Hughes's explanation that "the passenger-side door [of his car] . . . was still covered in old duct tape" to keep his son Walker from opening it while they were driving down the highway?[8] Or Josh Greenfeld's blunt description of the consequences of leaving his son unsupervised even for a moment: "Excrement in his pants, excrement on the bed, excrement smeared everywhere . . . loading up the washing machine, washing Noah down, changing the sheets and blankets, wiping the crap off the walls and the rug and the chairs, and doing all the shit-cleaning work our tired flesh has become heir to"?[9]

Or this memory of my life before Jonah's behaviors were medically stabilized: "When I try to remember what it was like to fight with my son, I see only hands: one wrapped over Jonah's fist, another under his jaw to keep him from biting, another untangling my hair from his fingers, one intercepting before he could yank another necklace off my neck . . . that's what it was, a blur of hands. I never had enough hands."[10] Because I am an autism parent-author also, of course, and this is exactly why I write about Jonah—to make sure he and his severely autistic peers are *seen*, even though it's so much easier to look away, to accept the intact mind as a sort of absolution that relieves us of the need to ask uncomfortable questions about dependency and obligation.

What if we didn't presume competence? Does that mean, by definition, that we presume *in*competence? Disability advocates are rightfully outraged by this alternative, haunted by the legacies of those who were historically deprived of appropriate educational, vocational, and social opportunities because their inability to speak—due to conditions like cerebral palsy, deafness, apraxia, or traumatic brain injury—was mistaken for severe cognitive impairment.

Jason Travers and Kevin Ayres point out, however, that the choice of presuming competence or incompetence represents a "false dichotomy." They propose that the only truly ethical alternative is "to refrain from presumptions entirely and instead insist on evidence to ascertain current functioning and alignment with current future environments (i.e., goals)." What kind of evidence? For these special education researchers, competency is a complex attribute that requires multiple and diverse types of information to measure, including standardized assessments; objective observation; data examining changes in functioning, if any, over time; and experimental analysis, in which environmental features are modified and resulting behaviors are tracked. Compared to the "wishful thinking" that characterizes the presumption of competence, Travers and Ayres argue, their evidence-based framework "is more rational, less dangerous, and better preserves the dignity of the person with the disability."[11]

This engagement with the material implications of the impaired mind aligns Travers and Ayres instrumentally with care ethics, which emerged in 1982 when psychologist Carol Gilligan challenged Lawrence Kohlberg's finding that boys scored higher than girls on his six-stage scale of moral development. It was not that boys were more sophisticated moral thinkers, Gilligan argued;

it was that boys and girls approached Kohlberg's ethical dilemmas using completely different frameworks. While boys applied a logic-based "ethic of justice"—to determine, for example, whether it was ethical for a man to break into a pharmacy and steal a prohibitively expensive drug that might save his dying wife—girls deployed an "ethic of care" that "reflects a cumulative knowledge of human relationships [and] evolves around a central insight, that self and other are interdependent."[12]

Subsequent scholars pushed back on Gilligan's identification of the ethic of care as a distinctively feminine "voice." In 1993, political scientist Joan Tronto pointed out that "what is lost in this association [between women and caring] is the reality of the complexity of caring, and the fact that caring is intertwined with virtually all aspects of life."[13] Agrees Eva Feder Kittay—who, inspired by her own cognitively impaired daughter, has written most extensively about care ethics in the context of intellectual disability: "We have discovered that men too are capable of caring for children and whomever [*sic*] is in need of care. . . . Once care is no longer regarded as an instinctual and a natural disposition found mostly in women, we can de-naturalize and de-gender care and understand it as a mode of moral conduct."[14]

Harvard physician and anthropologist Arthur Kleinman documents how he came to adopt this perspective while caring for his wife, Joan, through her decline and death from early-onset Alzheimer's disease in *The Soul of Care: The Moral Education of a Husband and a Doctor*. Before the onset of her illness, the Kleinmans adopted traditional gender roles in their marriage: Joan took primary responsibility for raising their children and supporting Arthur as he ascended to the highest echelons of academia. "I never made the bed, paid a bill, or tended to the house," Arthur remembers. "Joan played the role of primary carer in my life, and in the life of our family." But when their roles are reversed, he comes to a profound realization about this labor: "Care is not just a tool for getting through life by helping one another," he concludes. "It is also a necessary condition for living a life of purpose and passion. . . . Caring is what is morally and emotionally most at stake in human experience."[15]

What do we gain by considering service and supports for those with severe autism and other intellectual and developmental disabilities through the lens of care ethics? Most significantly, this paradigm offers a truly inclusive theory of human value that is completely detached from the criteria that have long been used to define personhood and citizenship, such as autonomy, cognition, or productivity. Instead, care ethicists emphasize our fundamental interconnectedness and mutual obligation. For Kittay, "the only universal and morally significant property that all humans possess is that we are all some mother's child," she writes. This indisputable commonality becomes the basis for a "moral equality" that locates care "at the center of our morality and politics."[16]

Key to this argument, however, is the recognition that "equality" is a fuzzy, polysemous concept that also allows Tronto to dispatch, with no hypocrisy, "the convenient fiction of human equality."[17] In other words, people with equal moral standing still differ wildly across the individual and social dimensions that shape life outcomes. This distinction, she argues, is glossed over in traditional moral theory—as well as, I would add, in much disability theory.

Given our history of devaluing the physically and intellectually disabled, of institutionalizing and sterilizing them, of routinely stripping them of all rights, this commitment to equality is completely understandable. But, as I hope I've demonstrated, the conflation of equality with the intact mind obscures critical *inequalities* in capacity, ability, and dependence. As Tronto elaborates, "Care is not an activity that occurs between equal and autonomous actors or objects, but between those who have needs and those who can provide for those needs."[18] Kittay, too, observes in care relationships what she calls "asymmetry in situation and power." For both these scholars, this is not something to be hushed or ignored, but an inherent part of the dependency we all experience more or less over the life span—whether due to infancy, dementia, psychosis, traumatic brain injury, or intellectual and developmental disability. Notes Kittay, the key question becomes how to negotiate these imbalances: "Care ethics then deals with our obligations and responsibilities in relationships of asymmetry."[19]

Critically, these conversations can't proceed without considering *both* sides of the care relationship. Care ethicists' attention to caregivers as well as recipients fills a huge gap in current disability discourse, which has been governed by what bioethicist Lisa Freitag calls "a cardinal rule that makes public optimism toward disability a requirement for the parent of a child with disabilities."[20] Although this rule is still strong in Disability Studies—one recent book labeled parents as "allies" or "obstacles" to their children based solely on their alignment with the goals of Disability Rights advocates[21]—an increasing number of voices are exposing the raw, messy, intimate labor required to care for loved ones with a range of conditions. Abby Maslin became her husband's nurse after he suffered a traumatic brain injury in a mugging, and had to learn "how to insert a long, plastic tube into T.C.'s trach and pull out the pink-tinged mucus that coats his lungs."[22] Kate Washington made her husband Brad's bed "lasagna-style, alternating fitted sheets and waterproof liners" because of the intense night sweats he suffered following his cancer diagnosis, which generated four loads of laundry every day.[23] Cynthia Lim's husband Perry was left almost helpless following a massive heart attack: "I squeezed toothpaste on his toothbrush and guided his hand to his mouth. He brushed lightly, then set the toothbrush on the counter. I followed up with more rigorous brushing. . . . I smeared shaving cream on my fingers, spread it on his cheeks. I placed the razor in his hand and he took a few feeble strokes. . . . He handed me the razor and I shaved the spots he missed."[24] Even more difficult than these physical tasks are the emotional sequelae of intense caregiving. All three writers elucidate the isolation, exhaustion, and frustration of caring for someone who can never be left alone—feelings very familiar to the parents of severely autistic children. As Maslin muses, "I don't know how to fulfill my duties, my loyalty to the person I love most, without losing myself in the process."[25]

Although good care often requires the prioritization of the needs of care recipients and the (at least temporary) deferral of the needs of caregivers, care ethicists recognize that this is not a tenable solution in the long term. Tronto advocates for "the need to keep a balance between the needs of caregivers and care-receivers."[26] Kittay in particular has written extensively about the need to support care work—which, in the United States, is overwhelmingly performed by women, immigrants, and members of racial and ethnic minorities. In her 1999 book *Love's Labor*, she calls for a social insurance program similar to workers' compensation or unemployment insurance that would ensure that all caregivers—both familial and professional—would receive meaningful compensation, including wages, health insurance, paid vacations, and housing.[27] With over 50 million American family members providing care every year,[28] care ethics invites us to imagine the infrastructure necessary to provide all who require it with the skilled, attentive, personal support we need to flourish.

Perhaps the most important lesson we can take from care ethics is that this support will look different for everyone. Both Tronto and Kittay argue that an individualized perspective is essential. "What is definitive about care," Tronto states, is "a perspective of taking the other's needs as the starting point for what must be done."[29] Similarly, Kittay emphasizes the duty of carers to "respond to this particular concrete other, not a generalized other," and identifies the aim of care as "*the flourishing (or minimally the well-being) of a person for his or her own sake, that is, not for the sake of the larger community or some abstract conception of goodness*" (emphasis in original).[30]

Yet this is exactly what drives contemporary disability policy: an abstract commitment to "inclusion" that has been weaponized against the intensive, specialized educational, vocational, and residential settings that may be required by those with challenging behaviors, or simply preferred by those seeking a community of peers. I have included chapters on the fight to eliminate 14(c) programs and guardianship, but I easily could have used other examples: the push to educate all children in inclusive classrooms; or the attack on residential settings that house more than four unrelated people as "isolating" and "segregating."[31]

Importantly, these narrow policy targets are unsupported by evidence. Although a common refrain from Neurodiversity proponents is that "research shows an overwhelming degree of support" for smaller, more dispersed and integrated settings,[32] the few studies that have attempted to address this question are badly flawed—most notably because they typically fail to control for severity of intellectual disability or degree of challenging behavior, key factors in determining the quality and intensity of necessary services.[33] A 2017 review of the literature by David Mandell, director of the Center for Mental Health Policy and Services Research at the University of Pennsylvania, concluded that "our decision-making regarding which types of placements to pay for and prioritize is based on values rather than data."[34]

Rather than a robust empirical base, at the core of this agenda is what I've (somewhat cheekily) called elsewhere "the reverse *Field of Dreams* fallacy"—the assertion that, "if we don't build it, they won't come."[35] In other words, according to staunch inclusion advocates, these types of disability-specific services are not really needed. But statistics suggest otherwise. As the number of facilities prepared to treat autistic individuals suffering from extreme aggression and self-injury has dropped, for example, families in crisis have been forced to turn to ill-equipped alternatives. A 2017 Kaiser Health News investigation found that the number of autistic individuals seen in emergency rooms doubled between 2009 and 2014, to almost 160,000 per year, where these patients may spend "weeks or even months . . . sometimes sedated, restrained or confined to mesh-tented beds,"[36] waiting for more appropriate placements—which might never come. In July 2021, twelve-year-old Emmett Tolis was admitted to the Children's Hospital of Philadelphia because his parents couldn't safely manage his dangerous behaviors. After four months of what his father described as "warehous[ing]," during which Emmett was routinely "strapped to his hospital bed," he was summarily discharged back to his family home. George Tolis told the *Philadelphia Inquirer* that, although he was "very happy that [Emmett's] going to be home," he was also "really terrified of what's going to happen."[37]

As I write this, in September 2022, the Tolis family is still waiting for a residential placement for Emmett. Importantly, this lack of support is not accidental, or an unintended consequence, or the result—like so many service disruptions—of COVID-era staffing shortages. It is, simply put, the intact mind in action. This historically contingent trope—shaped not by biology but by convergent discourses in psychoanalysis, cerebral palsy, and Disability

Rights, and amplified across five decades of autism parent memoirs—is the ideological driver of a Pennsylvania system that, as a result, has little to offer to those who need help most. And it's not just Pennsylvania—as we've seen, the influence of the intact mind can be seen in disability policy all over the country, at both state and federal levels.

* * *

I read more than eighty memoirs for this project, but my favorite wasn't actually written by a parent. *Boy Alone* tells the story of Noah Greenfeld—arguably "the most famous autistic child in America"[38] after his father wrote three books about him—from the perspective of his older brother, Karl Taro Greenfeld. Like Josh Greenfeld, Karl became a professional writer, and his lovely prose was certainly part of the appeal for me. But the real reason this one hit me harder than any other is an almost sixty-page chapter near the end of the book. Titled "2002," it describes Noah's "great breakthrough"[39]—how he finally emerged from autism and began speaking, listening, and, most critically, *understanding*; how he learned to cook, traveled to Europe and Asia, worked part-time as a proofreader for the local newspaper, and fell in love with a woman he ended up marrying.

I read in an increasing state of shock, filling the margins with exclamation points and question marks. Was it really possible that after inspiring the grimmest autism parent memoirs ever published, Noah Greenfeld would become the poster child for the intact mind? Was that degree of transformation truly possible for someone in his twenties? And of course, the thought that gripped me the entire time: *What about Jonah???*

Then I reached the next chapter, "Reality," which opens with this admission: "Noah is still alone. Noah never traveled to New York, Holland, or Hong Kong. He never reconnected with Latanya. Noah never spoke." He is, instead, "a man in torn, ragged clothes, banging his head against a concrete floor, scratching himself, spitting, pinching."[40]

I felt so angry reading that portrait of the real Noah, so manipulated. Why on earth had Greenfeld inserted this fantasy into a book that included the word "memoir" in the subtitle?

"I dreamed that happy outcome," he explains. "I imagined the life I wanted for me, for Noah, for my parents. I conjured it, as therapy, as a study in what if, as an attempted answer to the great question in our family: What if Noah could talk? What if Noah were normal? What if? What if?"[41]

This is why *Boy Alone* is powerful, for me. Because nothing else I've read gets to the heart of the issue: we can pretend the intact mind as much as we want.

We can, as Greenfeld does, imagine the exact words our loved one would say, or the outfit he would wear on his first date (for Noah, a polo shirt, jeans, and sneakers with Velcro straps). More broadly, we can pretend that *everyone* can live independently, make his own decisions, and hold competitive, minimum-wage employment. But—and this is the hardest, most painful truth I ever had to learn—that doesn't make it so. And if we base our system of supports and services for the autistic and intellectually disabled on pretend Noahs, and pretend Emmetts, and pretend Jonahs, we will always have a system that fails the real Noahs, the real Emmetts, the real Jonahs. Respecting the personhood of the severely autistic and intellectually disabled, maximizing their opportunities, and ensuring their lives are filled with joy and meaning requires honest conversations about the impaired mind, not pretending it away.

Notes

Introduction

1. Portia Iversen, *Strange Son: Two Mothers, Two Sons, and the Quest to Unlock the Hidden World of Autism* (New York: Riverhead Books, 2006), 74, 53, 55.
2. Judy Barron and Sean Barron, *There's a Boy in Here: A Mother and Her Son Tell the Story of His Emergence from Autism* (Arlington, TX: Future Horizons, 2002), 61.
3. Catherine Maurice, *Let Me Hear Your Voice: A Family's Triumph over Autism* (New York: Alfred A. Knopf, 1993), 82.
4. Cheri Florance, *Maverick Mind: A Mother's Story of Solving the Mystery of Her Unreachable, Unteachable, Silent Son* (New York: G. P. Putnam's Sons, 2004), 30.
5. Valerie Gilpeer and Emily Grodin, *I Have Been Buried under Years of Dust* (New York: William Morrow, 2021), 6.
6. Bryna Siegel, *The Politics of Autism* (Oxford: Oxford University Press, 2018), 204.
7. Rupert Isaacson, *The Horse Boy: A Memoir of Healing* (New York: Back Bay Books, 2009), 348.
8. Lori Ashley Taylor, *Dragonfly: A Daughter's Emergence from Autism* (New York: Skyhorse, 2018), 228.
9. Radiotimesteam, "Interview: Temple Grandin on Living with Autism," RadioTimes.com, https://www.radiotimes.com/movies/interview-temple-grandin-on-living-with-autism/.
10. Barry Neil Kaufman, *Son-Rise* (New York: Harper & Row, 1976), 42.
11. Maurice, *Let Me Hear Your Voice*, 80.
12. Robert Hughes, *Running with Walker* (London: Jessica Kingsley, 2003), 49.
13. Barron and Barron, *There's a Boy in Here*, viii–ix.
14. A note on language: there is much strife in the autism community over the use of person-first language (i.e., "child with autism," versus identify-first language, i.e., "autistic child"). Most of the parents of severely autistic children I know, including myself, care only that the language used to describe our children is respectful, and we see no meaningful difference between these iterations. But because many autistic adults dramatically prefer identity-first language, I primarily use it here.
15. Josh Greenfeld, *A Child Called Noah* (New York: Henry Holt, 1972), 180.
16. Hughes, *Running with Walker*, 235.
17. Leo Kanner, "Autistic Disturbances of Affective Contact," *Nervous Child: Journal of Psychopathology, Psychotherapy, Mental Hygiene, and Guidance of the Child* 2 (1943): 242.
18. Ka-Yuet Liu, Marissa King, and Peter S. Bearman, "Social Influence and the Autism Epidemic," *American Journal of Sociology* 115 (5): 1387–1434.
19. Kanner, "Autistic Disturbances of Affective Contact," 247.
20. Allison C. Carey, "Parents and Professionals: Parents' Reflections on Professionals, the Support System, and the Family in the Twentieth-Century United States," in *Disability Histories*, Susan Burch and Michael Rembis, eds. (Springfield: University of Illinois Press, 2014), 58.

21. Amanda Apgar, *The Disabled Child: Memoirs of a Normal Future* (Ann Arbor: University of Michigan Press, 2023), 3.
22. David T. Mitchell and Sharon L. Snyder, *Narrative Prosthesis: Disability and the Dependencies of Discourse* (Ann Arbor: University of Michigan Press, 2000), 166.
23. Alexa Ostrolenk, Baudouin Forgeot d'Arc, Patricia Jelenic, et al., "Hyperlexia: Systematic Review, Neurocognitive Modelling, and Outcome," *Neuroscience and Biobehavioral Reviews* 79 (2017): 139.
24. For more on the history of the Disability Rights Movement, see Richard K. Scotch, *From Good Will to Civil Rights: Transforming Federal Disability Policy* (Philadelphia: Temple University Press, 1984); Joseph P. Shapiro, *No Pity: People with Disabilities Forging a New Civil Rights Movement* (New York: Three Rivers Press, 1993); Doris Zames Fleischer and Frieda Zames, *The Disability Rights Movement: From Charity to Confrontation* (Philadelphia: Temple University Press, 2011); Lennard J. Davis, *Enabling Acts: The Hidden Story of How the Americans with Disabilities Act Gave the Largest US Minority Its Rights* (Boston: Beacon Press, 2016).
25. For more on the social model of disability, see Simi Linton, *Claiming Disability: Knowledge and Identity* (New York: New York University Press, 1998); Paul K. Longmore, *Why I Burned My Book: And Other Essays on Disability* (Philadelphia: Temple University Press, 2003); Tom Shakespeare, "The Social Model of Disability," in *The Disability Studies Reader*, 4th edition, Lennard J. Davis, ed. (New York: Routledge, 2013), 214–221.
26. Philip Ferguson, "The Social Construction of Mental Retardation," *Social Policy* 18, no. 1 (July 1987): 54.
27. For a full description of *Buck v. Bell*, see Paul A. Lombardo, *Three Generations, No Imbeciles: Eugenics, the Supreme Court, and* Buck v. Bell (Baltimore, MD: Johns Hopkins University Press, 2008) and Daniel Kevles, *In the Name of Eugenics: Genetics and the Uses of Human Heredity* (Cambridge, MA: Harvard University Press, 1985).
28. James Trent, *Inventing the Feeble Mind: A History of Mental Retardation in the United States* (Berkeley: University of California Press, 1994), 2.
29. Madeline C. Burghardt, *Broken: Institutions, Families, and the Construction of Intellectual Disability* (Montreal: McGill-Queen's University Press, 2018), 5.
30. Lombardo, *Three Generations, No Imbeciles*, 190.
31. Trent, *Inventing the Feeble Mind*, 80, 162, 270.
32. Steven Noll, *Feeble-Minded in Our Midst: Institutions for the Mentally Retarded in the South, 1900–1940* (Chapel Hill: University of North Carolina Press, 1995), 2. For more about the development and use of IQ tests, see Kevles, *In the Name of Eugenics*.
33. Patrick McDonagh, C. F. Goodey, and Tim Stainton, *Intellectual Disability: A Conceptual History, 1200–1900* (Manchester: Manchester University Press, 2018), 11.
34. Jim Sinclair, "Don't Mourn for Us," *Autonomy, the Critical Journal of Interdisciplinary Autism Studies* 1, no. 1 (October 2012): 3.
35. Judy Singer, *Odd People In: The Birth of Community amongst People on the "Autistic Spectrum": A Personal Exploration of a New Social Movement Based on Neurological Diversity*, a thesis presented to the faculty of Humanities and Social Sciences in partial fulfillment of the requirements for the degree of Bachelor of Arts Social Science (Honours), Faculty of Humanities and Social Science, University of Technology, Sydney, 1988, 12.
36. Steve Silberman, *NeuroTribes: The Legacy of Autism and the Future of Neurodiversity* (New York: Avery, 2015), 470.
37. Autistic Self-Advocacy Network, "About ASAN," https://autisticadvocacy.org/about-asan/.

38. Moheb Costandi, "Against Neurodiversity," *Aeon*, September 12, 2019. https://aeon.co/essays/why-the-neurodiversity-movement-has-become-harmful. See also Aviva Seigler, "Rebuttal: Dangerous World of Marginalizing Autism Parents," *Fierce Autie*, October 18, 2020, https://fierceautie.com/2020/10/18/rebuttal-dangerous-world-of-marginalizing-autism-parents/, and Cassandra Crosman, "The Autism Spectrum Is Not Binary," *In the Loop About Neurodiversity*, March 6, 2019, https://intheloopaboutneurodiversity.wordpress.com/2019/03/06/the-autism-spectrum-is-not-binary/, for just two of the many examples of this assertion.
39. Ferguson, "The Social Construction of Mental Retardation," 54.
40. Tom Shakespeare, *Disability Rights and Wrongs Revisited* (New York: Routledge, 2006), 96.
41. Mark Osteen, *Autism and Representation* (New York: Routledge, 2008), 4.
42. Stacy Clifford Simplican, *The Capacity Contract: Intellectual Disability and the Question of Citizenship* (Minneapolis: University of Minnesota Press), 11.
43. Eva Feder Kittay, *Learning from My Daughter: The Value and Care of Disabled Minds* (Oxford: Oxford University Press, 2019), 19.
44. Osteen, *Autism and Representation*, 299.
45. Michael Whelan, "Inspiration is Power: Voices of Information and Advocacy for the Reader of Autism Narratives," *Social Alternatives* 36, no. 4 (2017): 47.
46. Siegel, *The Politics of Autism*, 271.
47. James T. Fisher, "No Search, No Subject? Autism and the American Conversion Narrative," in *Autism and Representation*, Mark Osteen, ed. (New York: Routledge, 2008), 51, 62.
48. Hughes, *Running with Walker*, 110.
49. Annabel Stehli, *The Sound of a Miracle: A Child's Triumph over Autism* (New York: Doubleday, 1991).
50. Karyn Seroussi, *Unraveling the Mystery of Autism and Pervasive Developmental Disorder: A Mother's Story of Research and Recovery* (New York: Simon & Schuster, 2000).
51. G. Thomas Couser, *Signifying Bodies: Disability in Contemporary Life Writing* (Ann Arbor: University of Michigan Press, 2009), 5. For more on the archetypical role held by Down syndrome in the 1970s, see David Wright, *Downs: The History of a Disability* (Oxford: Oxford University Press, 2011), 174.
52. Clara Claiborne Park, *The Siege: The First Eight Years of an Autistic Child* (Boston: Little, Brown, 1967), 12.
53. Paul S. Appelbaum, "There are All Kinds of Rights," *The Hastings Center Report* 46, no. 2 (March–April 2016): inside back cover.

Chapter 1

1. Pearl S. Buck, *The Child Who Never Grew* (New York: John Day, 1950), 25.
2. Ibid., 35.
3. Ibid., 44.
4. Stanley Finger and Shawn E. Christ, "Pearl S. Buck and Phenylketonuria (PKU)," *Journal of the History of the Neurosciences* 13, no. 1 (2004): 45.
5. Buck, *The Child Who Never Grew*, 25.
6. Ibid., 25.
7. Ibid., 81.
8. Ibid., 83.

9. Maxine Garrison, *The Angel Spreads Her Wings: The Inspiration of* Angel Unaware *and the Influence of the Roy Rogers Family in the American Home* (Westwood, NJ: Fleming H. Revell, 1956), 14, 24.
10. Dale Evans Rogers, *Angel Unaware: A Touching Story of Love and Loss, 50th Anniversary Edition* (Grand Rapids, MI: Revell, 2004), 15.
11. Ibid., 24.
12. Ibid., 55.
13. Ibid., 85, 89.
14. Viviana A. Zelizer, *Pricing the Priceless Child* (New York: Basic Books, 1985), 11, 209.
15. John Gunther, *Death Be Not Proud: A Memoir* (New York: Harper & Row, 1949), 107.
16. Ibid., 45.
17. Buck, *The Child Who Never Grew*, 78–79.
18. Evans Rogers, *Angel Unaware*, 93.
19. Robert B. Edgerton, *The Cloak of Competence: Stigma in the Lives of the Mentally Retarded* (Berkeley: University of California Press, 1967), vii.
20. Peter L. Tyor and Leland V. Bell, *Caring for the Retarded in America: A History* (Westport, CT: Greenwood Press, 1984), x.
21. Nicole Rafter, "The Criminalization of Mental Retardation," in *Mental Retardation in America: A Historical Reader*, Steven Noll and James W. Trent, Jr., eds. (New York: New York University Press, 2004), 235.
22. Leila Zenderland, "The Parable of *The Kallikak Family:* Explaining the Meaning of Heredity in 1912," in *Mental Retardation in America*, 166.
23. Richard L. Dugdale, *The Jukes: A Study in Crime, Pauperism, Disease and Heredity* (New York: G. P. Putnam's Sons, 1877), 55.
24. Kevles, *In the Name of Eugenics*, 20. See also Lombardo, *Three Generations, No Imbeciles.*
25. Henry Herbert Goddard, *The Kallikak Family: A Study in the Heredity of Feeble-Mindedness* (New York: Macmillan, 1912), 29.
26. Noll and Trent, eds., *Mental Retardation in America*, 11.
27. J. David Smith and Michael L. Wehmeyer, "Who Was Deborah Kallikak?" *Intellectual and Developmental Disabilities* 50, no. 2 (2012): 169–178.
28. Samuel A. Kirk, Merle B. Karnes, and Winifred D. Kirk, *You and Your Retarded Child: A Manual for Parents of Retarded Children* (New York: Macmillan, 1955), 7.
29. Abraham Levinson, *The Mentally Retarded Child: A Guide for Parents* (New York: John Day, 1952), 29.
30. Katherine Castles, "'Nice, Average Americans': Postwar Parents' Groups and the Defense of the Normal Family," in *Mental Retardation in America*, 354.
31. Evans Rogers, *Angel Unaware.*
32. Buck, *The Child Who Never Grew*, 27, 33.
33. Lucille Stout, *I Reclaimed My Child: The Story of a Family into Which a Retarded Child Was Born* (Philadelphia: Chilton, 1959), 34.
34. Michael L. Wehmeyer and Robert L. Schalock, "The Parent Movement: Late Modern Times (1950 CE to 1980 CE)," in *The Story of Intellectual Disability: An Evolution of Meaning, Understanding, and Public Perception*, Michael L. Wehmeyer, ed. (Baltimore, MD: Paul H. Brookes, 2013), 188.
35. Stuart Murray, *Representing Autism: Culture, Narrative, Fascination* (Liverpool, UK: Liverpool University Press, 2008), 134.
36. Barron H. Lerner, *When Illness Goes Public: Celebrity Patients and How We Look at Medicine* (Baltimore, MD: Johns Hopkins University Press, 2006).

37. Ibid., 49.
38. Trent, *Inventing the Feeble Mind*, 234.
39. Kirk, Karnes, and Kirk, *You and Your Retarded Child*, 1.
40. Evans Rogers, *Angel Unaware*, 12.
41. John P. Frank, *My Son's Story* (New York: Alfred A. Knopf, 1952), 89.
42. Trent, *Inventing the Feeble Mind*, 233.
43. J. Norman Heard, *Hope through Doing* (New York: John Day, 1968), 184.
44. Charlotte D. Tucker, *Betty Lee: Care of Handicapped Children* (New York: Macmillan, 1954), 29.
45. Dorothy Garst Murray, *This Is Stevie's Story: A Mother's Story of Her Mentally Retarded Son* (Nashville, TN: Abingdon Press, 1956), 58.
46. Carvel Lee, *Tender Tyrant: The Story of a Mentally Retarded Child* (Minneapolis, MN: Augsburg, 1961), 6.
47. Horst Bickel, John Gerrard, and Evelyn M. Hickmans, "The Influence of Phenylalanine Intake on the Chemistry and Behaviour of a Phenylketonuric Child," *Acta Paediatrica* 43 (January 1954): 64–77.
48. Clemens E. Benda, *The Child with Mongolism (Congenital Acromicria)* (New York: Grune and Stratton, 1960), 205. For more on early theories of the etiology of Down syndrome, see Kate Brousseau, *Mongolism: A Study of the Physical and Mental Characteristics of Mongolian Imbeciles* (Baltimore, MD: Williams & Wilkins, 1928), Theodore H. Ingalls, "Etiology of Mongolism: Epidemiologic and Teratologic Implications," *American Journal of Diseases of Children* 74, no. 2 (1947): 147–165; David Wright, *Downs: The History of a Disability* (Oxford: Oxford University Press, 2011).
49. Leo Kanner, *A History of the Care and Study of the Mentally Retarded* (Springfield, IL: Charles C. Thomas, 1964), 133–134.
50. Sophia Gant, *"One of Those": The Progress of a Mongoloid Child* (New York: Pageant Press, 1957), 22.
51. B. R. Schmalzreid, Sr., *Sunshine: A Slow Miracle* (Boston, MA: Daughter of St. Paul, 1965), 67, 27.
52. Heard, *Hope Through Doing*, 148.
53. Pearl S. Buck, *The Gifts They Bring: Our Debt to the Mentally Retarded* (New York: John Day, 1965), 13, 48, 108, 131, 144, 146.
54. See, for example, Ian Brown, *The Boy in the Moon* (New York: St. Martin's Press, 2009), 182.
55. Nancy Roberts, *David* (Richmond, VA: John Knox Press, 1968), 52.
56. Martha Beck, *Expecting Adam: A True Story of Birth, Rebirth, and Everyday Magic* (New York: Three Rivers Press, 1999), 332.
57. Vicki Forman, *This Lovely Life: A Memoir of Premature Motherhood* (Boston: Mariner Books, 2009), 71.
58. Tucker, *Betty Lee*, 50.
59. Gant, *"One of Those,"* 12.
60. Schmalzried, *Sunshine*, 31.
61. Tucker, *Betty Lee*, 16.
62. Frank, *My Son's Story*, 58.
63. Clemens E. Benda, *Developmental Disorders of Mentation and Cerebral Palsies* (New York: Grune & Stratton, 1952), xv.
64. Marie Killilea, *Karen: A True Story Told by Her Mother* (New York: Open Road Integrated Media, 2018), 45, 34, 40.

65. Ibid., 45.
66. Ibid., 119, 38.
67. Earl R. Carlson, *Born That Way* (New York: John Day, 1941), 12.
68. Christy Brown, *My Left Foot* (London: Secker and Warburg, 1954), 15.
69. Joseph John Deacon, *Joey: An Unforgettable Story of Human Courage* (New York: Charles Scribner's Sons, 1974), 92.
70. Ruth Sienkiewicz-Mercer and Steven B. Kaplan, *I Raise My Eyes to Say Yes* (West Hartford, CT: Whole Health Books, 1989), 3, 8.
71. Nicola Schaefer, *Does She Know She's There?* (Markham, ON: Fitzhenry and Whiteside, 1999), 268.
72. Helene Brown, *Yesterday's Child* (New York: Signet, 1977), 3, 6, 42.
73. Sienkiewicz-Mercer and Kaplan, *I Raise My Eyes to Say Yes*, ix, xv.

Chapter 2

1. Technically, this is inaccurate. Jacques May's book *A Physician Looks at Psychiatry* was published in 1958. But, although May's project was inspired and informed by his experience as the father of autistic twins, his primary purpose—as evidenced by the title—was not to write a parent memoir but to leverage his medical expertise to castigate the field of psychiatry for its Freudian focus.
2. "Nobody/somebody memoirs" coined by Lorraine Adams, but quoted in G. Thomas Couser, "Introduction: Disability and Life Writing," *Journal of Literary & Cultural Disability Studies* 5, no. 3 (2011): 229.
3. Bernard Rimland, *Infantile Autism* (New York: Appleton-Century-Crofts, 1964), 18.
4. Leo Kanner, "Early Infantile Autism Revisited," *Psychiatry Digest* 29, no. 2 (February 1968): 24.
5. Stuart Murray, *Autism* (New York: Routledge, 2012), 57.
6. Centers for Disease Control and Prevention, "Facts about Developmental Disabilities," https://www.cdc.gov/ncbddd/developmentaldisabilities/facts.html.
7. Kanner, "Autistic Disturbances of Affective Contact," 247.
8. Leo Kanner, "Problems of Nosology and Psychodynamics of Early Infantile Autism," *Journal of Orthopsychiatry* 19, no. 3 (1949): 419; 416–426.
9. Heather E. Keith and Kenneth D. Keith, *Intellectual Disability: Ethics, Dehumanization, and a New Moral Community* (Malden, MA: Wiley Blackwell, 2013), 8.
10. Charles Mercier, *Sanity and Insanity* (London: Walter Scott, 1890), 287.
11. Ibid., 284.
12. William W. Ireland, *The Mental Affections of Children: Idiocy, Imbecility and Insanity* (London: J. & A. Churchill, 1898), 6.
13. Cynthia Lewiecki-Wilson, "Rethinking Rhetoric through Mental Disabilities," *Rhetoric Review* 22, no. 2 (2003): 157.
14. Margaret Price, "Defining Mental Disability," in *The Disability Studies Reader*, 4th edition, 304.
15. Gil Eyal, Brendan Hart, Emine Onculer, et al. *The Autism Matrix: The Social Origins of the Autism Epidemic* (Cambridge, UK: Polity Press, 2010), 214.
16. Ireland, *The Mental Affections of Children*, 273.
17. Alfred L. Baldwin, "Current Trends of Research in Child Development," in *Psychopathology of Childhood*, Paul H. Hoch and Joseph Zubin, eds. (New York: Grune and Stratton, 1955), 25.

18. Margarethe A. Ribble, "Disorganizing Factors of Infant Personality," *American Journal of Psychiatry* 98, no. 3 (1941): 459.
19. Beata Rank, "Adaptation of the Psychoanalytic Technique for the Treatment of Young Children with Atypical Development," *American Journal of Orthopsychiatry* 19, no. 1 (1949): 130, 132, 136, 138.
20. Frieda Fromm-Reichmann, "Notes on the Development of Treatment of Schizophrenics by Psychoanalytic Psychotherapy," *Psychiatry* 11, no. 3 (1948): 265.
21. Majia Holmer Nadesan, *Constructing Autism: Unravelling the "Truth" and Understanding the Social* (London: Routledge, 2005), 4.
22. Edward Dolnick, *Madness on the Couch: Blaming the Victim in the Heyday of Psychoanalysis* (New York: Simon & Schuster, 1998), 56.
23. Nadesan, *Constructing Autism*, 84.
24. Kathleen W. Jones, "'Mother Made Me Do It': Mother-Blaming and the Women of Child Guidance," in *"Bad" Mothers: The Politics of Blame in Twentieth-Century America,* Molly Ladd-Taylor and Lauri Umansky, eds. (New York: New York University Press, 1998), 104. For more on child guidance, see Kathleen W. Jones, *Taming the Troublesome Child: American Families, Child Guidance, and the Limits of Psychiatric Authority* (Cambridge, MA: Harvard University Press, 1999).
25. Quoted in Jones, " 'Mother Made Me Do It,' " 105.
26. John Neill, "Whatever Became of the Schizophrenogenic Mother?" *American Journal of Psychotherapy* XLIV, no. 4 (October 1990): 503.
27. Philip Wylie, *Generations of Vipers* (New York: Farrar & Rinehart, 1942), 215, 194, 206, 201.
28. Edward A. Strecker, *Their Mothers' Sons: The Psychiatrist Examines an American Problem* (Philadelphia: J. B. Lippincott, 1946), 31, 23.
29. Anne Harrington, "Mother Love and Mental Illness: An Emotional History," *Osiris* 31 (2016): 101.
30. Leo Kanner, *In Defense of Mothers: How to Bring Up Children in Spite of the More Zealous Psychologists* (Springfield, IL: Charles C. Thomas, 1941), 6.
31. Ibid., 131.
32. Ibid., 137.
33. Chloe Silverman, *Understanding Autism: Parents, Doctors, and the History of a Disorder* (Princeton, NJ: Princeton University Press, 2012), 32–33.
34. Kanner, "Autistic Disturbances of Affective Contact," 249, 217.
35. Bonnie Evans, *The Metamorphosis of Autism: A History of Child Development in Britain* (Manchester, UK: Manchester University Press, 2017.
36. Kanner, "Autistic Disturbances of Affective Contact," 242.
37. Ibid., 250.
38. Kanner, "Problems of Nosology," 425.
39. Leo Kanner, "To What Extent Is Early Infantile Autism Determined by Constitutional Inadequacies?" *Association for Research in Nervous and Mental Disease* 33, no. 1 (1954): 384, 383.
40. Leon Eisenberg and Leo Kanner, "Early Infantile Autism, 1943–1955," *American Psychiatry Association Research Report* 1 (1957): 561–562.
41. Silverman, *Understanding Autism*, 37.
42. Nadesan, *Constructing Autism*, 78.
43. John Donvan and Caren Zucker, *In a Different Key: The Story of Autism* (New York: Crown, 2016), 91.

44. Lauretta Bender, "The Development of a Schizophrenic Child Treated with Electric Convulsions at Three Years of Age," in *Emotional Problems of Early Childhood*, Gerald Caplan, ed. (New York: Basic Books, 1955), 425.
45. Lauretta Bender, *Psychopathology of Children with Organic Brain Disorders* (Springfield, IL: Charles C. Thomas, 1956), 43, 120.
46. Lauretta Bender, "Autism in Children with Mental Deficiency," *American Journal of Mental Deficiency* 64, no. 1 (January 1959): 84.
47. Mitzi Waltz, *Autism: A Social and Medical History* (Hampshire, UK: Palgrave Macmillan, 2013), 63.
48. J. Louise Despert, *The Emotionally Disturbed Child: Then and Now* (New York: Robert Brunner, 1965), 202.
49. Jordynn Jack, *Autism and Gender: From Refrigerator Mothers to Computer Geeks* (Urbana, IL: University of Chicago Press, 2014), 43.
50. John Bowlby, *Maternal Care and Mental Health: A Report Prepared on Behalf of the World Health Organization as a Contribution to the United Nations Programme for the Welfare of Homeless Children* (Geneva: World Health Organization, 1951), 11–12.
51. For more about Bowlby, ethology, and the development of attachment theory, see Frank C. P. van der Horst, *John Bowlby: From Psychoanalysis to Ethology* (West Sussex, UK: Wiley-Blackwell, 2011) and Marga Vicedo, *The Nature and Nurture of Love: Imprinting to Attachment in Cold War America* (Chicago: University of Chicago Press, 2013).
52. Deborah Blum, *Love at Goon Park* (Cambridge, MA: Perseus, 2002), 177, 232.
53. Lenny van Rosmalen, René van der Veer, and Frank C. P. van der Horst, "The Nature of Love: Harlow, Bowlby and Bettelheim on Affectionless Mothers," *History of Psychiatry* 31, no. 2 (2020): 230.
54. John Bowlby, *Attachment and Loss*, Vol. I: *Attachment* (New York: Basic Books, 1969), 345.
55. Nikolaas Tinbergen, "Ethology and Stress Diseases," *Science* 185, no. 4145 (July 5, 1974): 22.
56. Nikolaas Tinbergen and Elisabeth A. Tinbergen, *"Autistic" Children: New Hope for a Cure* (London; Boston; Sydney: George Allen & Unwin, 1983).
57. Harry F. Harlow and William T. McKinney, "Nonhuman Primates and Psychoses," *Journal of Autism and Childhood Schizophrenia* 1, no. 4 (1971): 371.
58. Uta Frith, "Review: *'Autistic' Children: New Hope for Cure*," *Psychological Medicine* 14 (1984): 461.
59. Bruno Bettelheim, *The Empty Fortress: Infantile Autism and the Birth of the Self* (New York: Free Press, 1967), 125.
60. Mira Rothenberg and Homer Page, "The Rebirth of Jonny," *Harper's Magazine* 220, no. 1317 (February 1, 1960): 57, 63.
61. Virginia M. Axline, *Dibs in Search of Self* (New York: Ballantine Books, 1964), vii.
62. Ibid., 80, 93.
63. Fisher, "No Search, No Subject?" 54.
64. Axline, *Dibs*, 30, 50, 219.
65. Waltz, *Autism*, 100.
66. Fisher, "No Search, No Subject?" 53.
67. Dolnick, *Madness on the Couch*, 205.
68. Park, *The Siege*, 89.
69. Marga Vicedo, *Intelligent Love: The Story of Clara Park, Her Autistic Daughter, and the Myth of the Refrigerator Mother* (Boston: Beacon Press, 2021), 92.
70. Park, *The Siege*, 125.

71. Carey, "Parents and Professionals," 59.
72. Park, *The Siege*, 131.
73. Waltz, *Autism*, 111.
74. Adam Feinstein, *A History of Autism: Conversations with the Pioneers* (West Sussex, UK: John Wiley & Sons, 2010), 100.
75. Vicedo, *Intelligent Love*, 137.
76. Ibid., 275.
77. Margaret S. Mahler, Fred Pine, and Anni Bergman, *The Psychological Birth of the Human Infant* (New York: Basic Books, 1975), 11.
78. Park, *The Siege*, 34.
79. Despert, *The Emotionally Disturbed Child*, 194.
80. Axline, *Dibs*, 22.
81. Pollak, *The Creation of Dr. B.*, 276.
82. Park, *The Siege*, 12, 79, 119, 133.
83. Ibid., 161.
84. Ibid., 271.
85. Vicedo, *Intelligent Love*, 125–126.
86. Jack, *Autism and Gender*, 55.
87. Ibid., 272.
88. Park, *The Siege*, 169.
89. Ibid., 42.
90. Kanner, "Autistic Disturbances of Affective Contact," 226, 231, 230.
91. Ibid., 261.
92. Ibid., 270.
93. Park, *The Siege*, 85.
94. Vicedo, *Intelligent Love*, 125.
95. Rank, "Adaptation of the Psychoanalytic Technique," 133.
96. Frances Tustin, *Autism and Childhood Psychosis* (London: Hogarth, 1972), 104.
97. Dolnick, *Madness on the Couch*, 192.
98. Park, *The Siege*, 110.
99. Joan Martin Hundley, *The Small Outsider: The Story of an Autistic Child* (New York: St. Martin's Press, 1971), 35.
100. Ibid., 145–147.
101. Greenfeld, *A Child Called Noah*, 139.
102. Ibid., 179, 140, 64, 98.
103. Ibid., 4, 165, 141.
104. Josh Greenfeld, *A Place for Noah* (New York: Holt, Rinehart and Winston, 1978), 2.
105. James Copeland, with Jack Hodges, *For the Love of Ann* (New York: Ballantine Books, 1973), 12, 15.
106. Ibid., 32.
107. Ibid., 135, 34.
108. Ibid., 38.
109. Ibid., 119, 149.
110. Kaufman, *Son-Rise*, 23, 48.
111. Ibid., 40, 49.
112. Ibid., 36, 48, 72, 129, 85.
113. Ibid., 148, 150.

114. Osteen, *Autism and Representation*, 18.
115. Michael Rutter, "Medical Aspects of the Education of Psychotic (Autistic) Children," in *Some Approaches to Teaching Autistic Children: A Collection of Papers*, P.T.B. Weston, ed. (Oxford: Pergamon Press, 1965), 66.

Chapter 3

1. Julie Rak, *Boom! Manufacturing Memoir for the Popular Market* (Waterloo, ON: Wilfrid Laurier University Press, 2013), 9.
2. Claire Laurier Decoteau and Meghan Daniel, "Scientific Hegemony and the Field of Autism," *American Sociological Review* 85, no. 3 (June 2020): 11.
3. Stuart Murray, *Representing Autism*, 85. For more about the influence of *Rain Man*, see also Anthony D. Baker, "Recognizing Jake: Contending with Formulaic and Spectacularized Representations of Autism in Film," in *Autism and Representation*, Mark Osteen, ed. (New York: Routledge, 2008), 229–243.
4. Rimland, *Infantile Autism*, 93.
5. Rutter, "Medical Aspects of the Education of Psychotic (Autistic) Children," 68.
6. Lorna Wing, *Children Apart: Autistic Children and Their Families* (British Medical Association in conjunction with the National Association for Mental Health, 1970), 21.
7. Richard J. Schain and Daniel X. Freedman, "Studies on 5-Hydroxyindole Metabolism in Autistic and Other Mentally Retarded Children," *Journal of Pediatrics* 58 (March 1961): 315–320.
8. C. Hutt, S. J. Hutt, D. Lee, and C. Ounsted, "Arousal and Childhood Autism," *Nature, London* 204 (1964): 908–909.
9. M. Rutter, D. Greenfeld, and L. Lockyer, "A Five to Fifteen-Year Follow-Up Study of Infantile Psychosis," *British Journal of Psychiatry* 113 (1967): 1183–1199.
10. Eric Schopler, "Parents of Autistic Children as Scapegoats," *Journal of Contemporary Psychotherapy* 4, no. 1 (Winter 1971): 20.
11. Donvan and Zucker, *A Different Key*, 93.
12. Frances Tustin, *Autistic States in Children* (London: Routledge, 1992), 11.
13. Annabel Stehli, *The Sound of a Miracle* (NY: Doubleday, 1990), 26, 29.
14. Barron, *There's a Boy in Here*, 110.
15. Jane Taylor McDonnell, *News from the Border: A Mother's Memoir of Her Autistic Son* (New York: Ticknor & Fields, 1993), 135.
16. For a detailed history of Bettelheim's life, see Pollak, *The Creation of Dr. B.*
17. Stehli, *The Sound of a Miracle*, 26.
18. Patricia Stacey, *The Boy Who Loved Windows: Opening the Heart and Mind of a Child Threatened with Autism* (Cambridge, MA: Da Capo Press, 2003), 117.
19. Quoted in Stehli, *The Sound of a Miracle*, 26.
20. Eyal et al., *The Autism Matrix*, 167–168.
21. Silverman, *Understanding Autism*, 114–115.
22. Wing, *Children Apart*, 17.
23. Marian K. DeMyer, *Parents and Children in Autism* (New York: John Wiley & Sons, 1979), 128, xii.
24. Charles Hart, *Without Reason: A Family Copes with Two Generations of Autism* (New York: Harper & Row, 1989), 76.

25. Barron, *There's a Boy in Here*, 171.
26. Florance, *Maverick Mind*, 102.
27. Marcia Hinds, *I Know You're in There: Winning Our War against Autism* (New York: Skyhorse, 2020), xxi, 66.
28. Susan Levin, *Unlocked: A Family Emerging from the Shadows of Autism* (New York: Skyhorse, 2015), xiii.
29. Florance, *Maverick Mind*, 233.
30. Jenny McCarthy, *Louder than Words: A Mother's Journey in Healing Autism* (New York: Dutton, 2007), 173.
31. Bill Davis, *Breaking Autism's Barriers: A Father's Story* (London: Jessica Kingsley, 2001), 375, 356, 306.
32. Paul Starr, *The Social Transformation of American Medicine* (New York: Basic Books, 1982), 391.
33. Tom Nichols, *The Death of Expertise: The Campaign against Established Knowledge and Why It Matters* (Oxford: Oxford University Press, 2017), xi.
34. Hinds, *I Know You're In There*, 57.
35. Stehli, *The Sound of a Miracle*, 56.
36. Charlotte Moore, *George & Sam: Two Boys, One Family, and Autism* (New York: St. Martin's Griffin, 2004), 278.
37. McDonnell, *News from the Border*, 110.
38. Elizabeth C. Evans, *Physiognomics in the Ancient World* (Philadelphia, PA: American Philosophical Society, 1969), 5.
39. Simon Jarrett, *Those They Called Idiots: The Idea of the Disabled Mind from 1700 to the Present Day* (London: Reaktion Books, 2020), 50, 72.
40. Mitchell and Snyder, *Narrative Prosthesis*, 60.
41. Moore, *George & Sam*, 136, 279.
42. Copeland, *For the Love of Ann*, 3.
43. Hart, *Without Reason*, 59.
44. Hughes, *Running with Walker*, 38.
45. Davis, *Breaking Autism's Barriers*, 33.
46. Beate Hermelin, *Bright Splinters of the Mind: A Personal Story of Research with Autistic Savants* (London: Jessica Kingsley, 2001), 17.
47. Murray, *Representing Autism*, 14.
48. Lorna Wing, "Asperger's Syndrome: A Clinical Account," *Psychological Medicine* 11 (1981): 115–129.
49. Silberman, *NeuroTribes*, 163.
50. Edith Sheffer, *Asperger's Children: The Origins of Autism in Nazi Vienna* (New York: W. W. Norton, 2018), 60.
51. Lorna Wing, "Reflections on Opening Pandora's Box," *Journal of Autism and Developmental Disorders* 35, no. 2 (April 2005): 198.
52. Lorna Wing, "Severe Impairments of Social Interaction and Associated Abnormalities in Children: Epidemiology and Classification," *Journal of Autism and Developmental Disorders* 9, no. 1 (1979): 11–29.
53. Christopher Gillberg and Lorna Wing, "Autism: Not an Extremely Rare Disorder," *Acta Psychiatrica* 99 (1999): 399.
54. Wing, "Reflections on Opening Pandora's Box," 197.
55. Hinds, *I Know You're in There*, 90.

56. Davis, *Breaking Autism's Barriers*, 36.
57. Susan Folstein and Michael Rutter, "Infantile Autism: A Genetic Study of 21 Twin Pairs," *Journal of Child Psychology and Psychiatry* 18, no. 4 (1977): 297–321.
58. Silverman, *Understanding Autism*, 44.
59. Hart, *Without Reason*, 94.
60. Zachary Warren, Jeremy Veenstra-VanderWeele, Wendy Stone, et al., *Therapies for Children with Autism Spectrum Disorders: Comparative Effectiveness Review No. 26* (Rockville, MD: Agency for Healthcare Research and Quality, 2011).
61. O. Ivar Lovaas, "Behavioral Treatment and Normal Educational and Intellectual Functioning in Young Autistic Children," *Journal of Consulting and Clinical Psychology* 55, no. 1 (1987): 3.
62. Maurice, *Let Me Hear Your Voice*, 80.
63. Carol Johnson and Julia Crowder, *Autism: From Tragedy to Triumph* (Boston, MA: Branden, 1994), 41, 70, 51.
64. Maurice, *Let Me Hear Your Voice*, 215, 290.
65. Johnson and Crowder, *Autism*, 177, 182.
66. Florance, *Maverick Mind*.
67. Stacey, *The Boy Who Loved Windows*.
68. McCarthy, *Louder than Words*.
69. Facilitated communication is the subject of Chapter 6; examples of memoirs include Iverson, *Strange Son*; Handley, *Underestimated*; Goddard and Goddard, *I Am Intelligent*; Gilpeer and Grodin, *I Have Been Buried under Years of Dust*; Hobson and Hobson, *I'm So Glad You Found Me in Here*; Savarese, *Reasonable People*; Bonker and Breen, *I Am in Here*; Martin, *Out of Silence*; Higashida, *The Reason I Jump*; Kedar, *Ido in Autismland*; and Tino, *The Autistic Mind Finally Speaks* (see Chapter 6 for full details).
70. Isaacson, *The Horse Boy*.
71. Iversen, *Strange Son*. For the history of genetic research in autism, see Jennifer S. Singh, *Multiple Autisms: Spectrums of Advocacy and Genomic Science* (Minneapolis: University of Minnesota Press, 2016).
72. Hinds, *I Know You're in There*.
73. Levin, *Unlocked*.
74. Levin, *Unlocked*, 8.
75. Isaacson, *The Horse Boy*, 315.
76. Connie Anderson, J. Kiely Law, Amy Daniels, et al., "Occurrence and Family Impact of Elopement in Children with Autism Spectrum Disorders," *Pediatrics* 130, no. 5 (November 1, 2012): 870.
77. Hinds, *I Know You're in There*, 30.
78. Taylor, *Dragonfly*, 12.
79. Maurice, *Let Me Hear Your Voice*, 33.
80. Florance, *Maverick Mind*, 12.
81. Maurice, *Let Me Hear Your Voice*, 40.
82. McCarthy, *Louder than Words*, 58.
83. Barron and Barron, *There's a Boy in Here*, 17.
84. Levin, *Unlocked*, 326.
85. Florance, *Maverick Mind*, 30.
86. Barron and Barron, *There's a Boy in Here*, 61.
87. Hinds, *I Know You're In There*, 52, 5.

88. Maurice, *Let Me Hear Your Voice*, 81–82.
89. Davis, *Breaking Autism's Barriers*, 163.
90. Hughes, *Running with Walker*, 210, 178.
91. Hughes, *Running with Walker*, 234.
92. Davis, *Breaking Autism's Barriers*, 384.
93. Hughes, *Running with Walker*, 196.
94. Hughes, *Running with Walker*, 234.
95. Davis, *Breaking Autism's Barriers*, 161.
96. Moore, *George & Sam*, 136.
97. Whitney Ellenby, *Autism Uncensored: Pulling Back the Curtain* (Virginia Beach, VA: Köehlerbooks, 2017), 13.
98. Murray, *Representing Autism*, 157.
99. Amy S. F. Lutz, *Each Day I Like It Better: Autism, ECT, and the Treatment of Our Most Impaired Children* (Nashville, TN: Vanderbilt University Press, 2014).
100. Catherine Lord, Eva Petkova, Vanessa Hus, et al., "A Multisite Study of the Clinical Diagnosis of Different Autism Spectrum Disorders," *Archives of General Psychiatry* 69, no. 3 (March 2012): 306–313.
101. Barron and Barron, *There's a Boy in Here*, 264.
102. Johnson and Crowder, *Autism: From Tragedy to Triumph*, 7.
103. Hinds, *I Know You're in There*, xv.
104. Aly Weisman, "Jenny McCarthy Slams 'Irresponsible' Rumor Her Son Was Misdiagnosed with Autism," *Business Insider*, January 6, 2014, https://www.businessinsider.com/jenny-mccarthy-slams-rumors-her-son-was-misdiagnosed-with-autism-2014-1.
105. Michael Rutter, "Autistic Children: Infancy to Adulthood," *Seminars in Psychiatry* 2 (1970): 435.
106. Molly Helt, Elizabeth Kelley, Marcel Kinsbourne, et al., "Can Children with Autism Recover? If So, How?" *Neuropsychology Review* 18 (2008): 339.
107. Deborah K. Anderson, Jessie W. Liang, and Catherine Lord, "Predicting Young Adult Outcome among More and Less Cognitively Able Individuals with Autism Spectrum Disorders," *The Journal of Child Psychology and Psychiatry* 55, no. 5 (2014): 485–494.
108. Helt et al., "Can Children with Autism Recover?," 349.
109. Alyssa J. Orinstein, Molly Helt, Eva Troyb, et al., "Intervention History of Children and Adolescents with High-Functioning Autism and Optimal Outcomes," *Journal of Developmental & Behavioral Pediatrics* 35, no. 4 (May 2014): 252.
110. Amy Sousa, "From Refrigerator Mothers to Warrior-Heroes: The Cultural Identity Transformation of Mothers Raising Children with Intellectual Disabilities," *Symbolic Interaction* 34, no. 2 (2011): 220, 235.
111. McCarthy, *Louder than Words*, 138.
112. Davis, *Breaking Autism's Barriers*, 288.
113. Levin, *Unlocked*, 325.
114. Taylor, *Dragonfly*, 155.
115. Clara Claiborne Park, *Exiting Nirvana: A Daughter's Life with Autism* (Boston, MA: Back Bay Books, 2001), 10.
116. Park, *Exiting Nirvana*, 24.
117. Ibid., 114.
118. Ibid., 53.
119. Ibid., 83.

120. Ellen Herman, "The Siege: The First Eight Years of an Autistic Child, 1967," The Autism History Project, https://blogs.uoregon.edu/autismhistoryproject/topics/the-siege-1967/.
121. Vicedo, *Intelligent Love*, 137.
122. Murray, *Representing Autism*, 175.
123. Ralph Savarese, *Reasonable People: A Memoir of Autism & Adoption* (New York: Other Press, 2007), xviii.
124. K. Tilden Frost, "I Don't Need or Want Your Autism Awareness," Geek Mom, April 6, 2018, https://geekmom.com/2018/04/i-dont-need-or-want-your-autism-awareness/.
125. Patrick Dwyer, Jacalyn G. Ryan, Zachary J. Williams, and Dena L. Gassner, "First Do No Harm: Suggestions Regarding Respectful Autism Language," *Pediatrics* 149, no. s4 (April 2022): s1, https://publications-aap-org.proxy.library.upenn.edu/pediatrics/article/149/Supplement%204/e2020049437N/185653/First-Do-No-Harm-Suggestions-Regarding-Respectful?autologincheck=redirected. See also Kristen Bottema-Beutel, Steven K. Kapp, Jessica Nina Lester, et al., "Avoiding Ableist Language: Suggestions for Autism Researchers," *Autism in Adulthood* 3, no. 1 (2021): 18–29, https://www-liebertpub-com.proxy.library.upenn.edu/doi/epdf/10.1089/aut.2020.0014. For a response I coauthored, see Alison Singer, Amy Lutz, Jill Escher, and Alycia Halladay, "A Full Semantic Toolbox Is Essential for Autism Research and Practice to Thrive," *Autism Research* 16 (2023): 497–501. https://onlinelibrary.wiley.com/doi/epdf/10.1002/aur.2876.

Chapter 4

1. A note on terminology: my interlocutors repeatedly told me that they no longer use the term "sheltered workshops," because it evokes images that advocates argue are dated and inaccurate—disabled adults forced to spend their days in dim warehouses, engaged in meaningless, repetitive labor, like sorting beads by color, only for them to be dumped into a bin to be re-sorted the next day. To honor their preferences, I refer to such programs by their regulatory classification, 14(c).
2. Andrea Zuber and Julia Burkstaller, "Letter to Members of the Senate Human Services Reform Finance and Policy Committee," November 10, 2021, https://www.senate.mn/committees/2021-2022/3096_Committee_on_Human_Services_Reform_Finance_and_Policy/The%20Arc%20Minnesota%20Subminimum%20Wage%20Written%20Testimo New York%2011.10.21.pdf.
3. John Wayne Barker, "Sameness," Bark's Bytes, Blog of Merrick, Inc., November 9, 2021, https://merrickinc.org/barks-bytes/barks-bytes-43-sameness/.
4. U.S. Commission on Civil Rights, "Subminimum Wages: Impacts on the Civil Rights of People with Disabilities," September 2020, viii, https://www.usccr.gov/files/2020/2020-09-17-Subminimum-Wages-Report.pdf.
5. Ibid., 230.
6. Carol Glazer, "Let's Stop Cheating the Disabled," National Organization on Disability, August 20, 2018, https://www.nod.org/lets-stop-cheating-the-disabled/.
7. Disability Rights Texas, "Living on a Dime and Left Behind: How a Depression-Era Labor Law Cheats Texas Workers with Disabilities," July 12, 2016, https://media.disabilityrightstx.org/wp-content/uploads/2018/10/22172109/Submin_Wage_Sheltered_Workshop_WHITE_PAPER_07_12_16_FINAL.pdf.

8. Office of Disability Policy, U.S. Department of Labor, "Defining Employment First," https://www.dol.gov/agencies/odep/initiatives/employment-first.
9. U.S. Commission on Civil Rights, "Subminimum Wages," 23, 28, 71.
10. National Disability Rights Network, "Segregated and Exploited: The Failure of the Disability Service System to Provide Quality Work," January 2011, 26, https://www.ndrn.org/wp-content/uploads/2019/03/Segregated-and-Exploited.pdf.
11. U.S. Commission on Civil Rights, "Subminimum Wages," 27
12. Nathan Nelson, *Workshops for the Handicapped in the United States: An Historical and Developmental Perspective* (Springfield, IL: Charles C. Thomas, 1971), 7.
13. U.S. Commission on Civil Rights, "Subminimum Wages," 60.
14. Ibid., xiii.
15. Interview with Lori Schluttenhofer, January 6, 2022.
16. Names of disabled individuals and family members have been changed to protect privacy.
17. Interview with Laura Johnson, January 3, 2022.
18. A. G. Crocker, C. Mercier, and Y. Lachapelle et al., "Prevalence and Types of Aggressive Behaviour among Adults with Intellectual Disabilities," *Journal of Intellectual Disability Research* 50 (September 2006): 652.
19. Micah O. Mazurek, Stephen M. Kanne, and Ericka L. Wodka, "Physical Aggression in Children and Adolescents with Autism Spectrum Disorders," *Research in Autism Spectrum Disorders* 7, no. 3 (March 2013): 455; 455–465.
20. Interview with John Wayne Barker, January 5, 2022.
21. Stephen Stafford, "Nothing Less than the Minimum: People with Disabilities Should Not Earn Less than Minimum Wage," *University of Cincinnati Law Review* (December 27, 2021), https://uclawreview.org/2021/12/27/nothing-less-than-the-minimum-people-with-disabilities-should-not-earn-less-than-minimum-wage/.
22. U.S. Commission on Civil Rights, "Subminimum Wages," 80.
23. Center for Health Care Strategies, "Trends and Challenges in Publicly-Financed Care for Individuals with Intellectual and Developmental Disabilities," September 2012, http://www.chcs.org/media/IDD_Service_Delivery_Systems_082812.pdf, 17.
24. U.S. Commission on Civil Rights, "Subminimum Wages," 251.
25. Milken Institute School of Public Health, Department of Health Policy & Management, George Washington University, "Transitions: A Case Study of the Conversion from Sheltered Workshops to Integrated Employment in Maine," 2015, https://docplayer.net/33593240-Transitions-a-case-study-of-the-conversion-from-sheltered-workshops-to-integrated-employment-in-maine.html, 7, 12.
26. Scott Spreat and James William Conroy, "Longitudinal Investigation of Vocational Engagement," *Journal of Policy and Practice in Intellectual Disabilities* 12, no. 4 (December 2015): 266–271. Importantly, age was not correlated to employment status in this sample, but adaptive behavior was. In other words, those with the most significant functional and behavioral limitations were the least likely to hold minimum-wage jobs.
27. U.S. Commission on Civil Rights, "Subminimum Wages," 47.
28. Ibid., xii, accompanying letter to Trump, Pence, and Pelosi.
29. U.S. Commission on Civil Rights, "Subminimum Wages," 4–5.
30. National Disability Rights Network, "Segregated and Exploited," 28.
31. Ibid., 3.
32. Ibid., 24, 16, 42.

33. Barbara Ehrenreich, *Nickel and Dimed: On (Not) Getting by in America* (New York: Metropolitan Books, 2001), 117, 220.
34. Disability Rights Network, "Segregated and Exploited," 24.
35. Michelle Murphy, *The Economization of Life* (Durham, NC: Duke University Press, 2017), 6.
36. Ibid., 6, 115.
37. Ari Ne'eman, "(Almost) Everything You Need to Know about Sheltered Workshops: Part 2 of 2," *Sometimes a Lion* (September 26, 2015), https://arineeman.com/2015/09/26/sheltered-workshops-part-2/. The average hourly rate of 14(c) employees is actually $3.34/hour, according to the UCCR report.
38. Sarah F. Rose, *No Right to Be Idle: The Invention of Disability, 1840s–1930s* (Chapel Hill: University of North Carolina Press, 2017), 10.
39. Fleischer and Zames, *The Disability Rights Movement*, 5–7.
40. Paul K. Longmore and David Goldberger, "The League of the Physically Handicapped and the Great Depression: A Case Study in the New Disability History," *The Journal of American History* 87, no. 3 (December 2000): 904.
41. League of the Physically Handicapped, "Thesis on Conditions of Physically Handicapped," August 1936, J. Paul Leonard Library Digital Collections, UARC_0145, http://digital-collections.library.sfsu.edu/digital/collection/p16737coll2/id/994/.
42. Longmore, *Why I Burned My Book*, 258.
43. Jasbir Puar, *The Right to Maim: Debility, Capacity, Disability* (Durham, NC: Duke University Press, 2017), 22.
44. David T. Mitchell with Sharon L. Snyder, *The Biopolitics of Disability: Neoliberalism, Ablenationalism, and Peripheral Embodiment* (Ann Arbor: University of Michigan Press, 2015), 5, 13.
45. U.S. Commission on Civil Rights, "Subminimum Wages," 251.
46. Matt London, "Geraldo: The Story 'Branded on My Soul' That Caused a Revolution," *Fox News*, January 21, 2020, foxnews.com/media/Geraldo-willowbrook-branded-my-soul-fox-nation.
47. Dan Barry, "The 'Boys' in the Bunkhouse: Toil, Abuse and Endurance in the Heartland," *New York Times*, March 9, 2014, https://www.New Yorktimes.com/interactive/2014/03/09/us/the-boys-in-the-bunkhouse.html.
48. Ralph Fevre, Amanda Robinson, and Duncan Lewis et al., "The Ill-Treatment of Employees with Disabilities in British Workplaces," *Work, Employment and Society* 27, no. 2 (2013): 297.
49. U.S. Commission on Civil Rights, "Subminimum Wages," 18–19.
50. *Olmstead v. L.C.* (1999), https://supreme.justia.com/cases/federal/us/527/581/.
51. Shapiro, *No Pity*, 102.
52. Sara Nović, "The Hearing World Must Stop Forcing Deaf Culture to Assimilate," *NBC News*, October 20, 2017, https://www.nbcnews.com/think/opinion/hearing-world-must-stop-forcing-deaf-culture-assimilate-ncna812461.
53. Jan Branson and Don Miller, "Sign Language, the Deaf and the Epistemic Violence of Mainstreaming," *Language and Education* 7, no. 1 (1993): 21.
54. U.S. Commission on Civil Rights, "Subminimum Wages," 265, 266.
55. Ehrenreich, *Nickel and Dimed*, 76.
56. Interview with Lori Schluttenhofer, January 6, 2022.
57. U.S. Commission on Civil Rights, "Subminimum Wages," 266.
58. Autistic Self-Advocacy Network, Self Advocates Becoming Empowered, and the National Youth Leadership Network, "Keeping the Promise: Self Advocates Defining the Meaning of

Community Living," accessed January 28, 2022, https://autisticadvocacy.org/wp-content/uploads/2012/02/KeepingthePromise-SelfAdvocatesDefiningtheMeaningofCommunity.pdf, 6.
59. Ibid., 3.

Chapter 5

1. Robert Dinerstein, "Implementing Legal Capacity under Article 12 of the UN Convention on the Rights of Persons with Disabilities: The Difficult Road from Guardianship to Supported Decision Making," *Human Rights Brief* 19, no. 2 (2012): 8–9.
2. National Council on Disability, *Beyond Guardianship: Toward Alternatives That Promote Greater Self-Determination*, March 22, 2018, 42, https://ncd.gov/publications/2018/beyond-guardianship-toward-alternatives https://ncd.gov/sites/default/files/NCD_Guardianship_Report_Accessible.pdf.
3. United Nations, World Autism Day, http://webtv.un.org/search/toward-autonomy-and-self-determination-world-autism-awareness-day-2017/5380816054001?term=world%20autism%20awareness%20day%202017.
4. SARTAC, "The Process of Terminating Guardianship Using Supported Decision Making," April 27, 2020, https://www.youtube.com/watch?v=PmWAZpItZ6Q.
5. Center for Public Representation, "U.S. Supported Decision-Making Laws," https://supporteddecisions.org/resources-on-sdm/state-supported-decision-making-laws-and-court-decisions/.
6. National Council on Disability, *Beyond Guardianship*, 54.
7. Piers Gooding, *A New Era for Mental Health Law and Policy: Supported Decision-Making and the UN Convention on the Rights of Persons with Disabilities* (Cambridge: Cambridge University Press, 2017), 22.
8. Eliza Buhrer, "Mental Competency Inquisitions from Medieval England (ca. late 12th c.–early 15th c.)," in *Medieval Disability Sourcebook*, Cameron Hunt McNabb, ed. (Santa Barbara, CA: Punctum Books, 2020), 56.
9. Kim E. Nielsen, "Property, Disability, and the Making of the Incompetent Citizen in the United States, 1860s–1940s," in *Disability Histories*, Susan Burch and Michael Rembis, eds. (Urbana: University of Illinois Press, 2014), 308–320.
10. Barry B. Swadron, *Mental Retardation—the Law—Guardianship* (Toronto, ON: National Institute on Mental Retardation, 1972), 186.
11. Shapiro, *No Pity*, 51–52. For more about the Disability Rights movement, see also Fleischer and Zames, *The Disability Rights Movement*.
12. Jae Kennedy, Simi Litvak, and Hale Zukas, "Independent Living and Personal Assistance Services: The Research, Training and Technical Assistance Programs at the World Institute on Disability," *Office of Special Education and Rehabilitation Services* 3 (1994): 43.
13. The President's Panel on Mental Retardation, "Report of the Task Force on Law," January, 1963, https://mn.gov/mnddc/parallels2/pdf/60s/63/63-ROT-PPMR.pdf.
14. Jennifer J. Monthie, "The Myth of Liberty and Justice for All: Guardianship in New York State," *Albany Law Review* 80, no. 3 (2017): 3.
15. Quoted in Swadron, *Mental Retardation*, 185.
16. United Nations, "Declaration on the Rights of Mentally Retarded Persons," December 20, 1971, https://www.ohchr.org/en/instruments-mechanisms/instruments/declaration-rights-mentally-retarded-persons.

17. Robert Perske, "The Dignity of Risk and the Mentally Retarded," *Mental Retardation* 10, no. 1 (1972): 26.
18. Wolf Wolfensberger, Bengt Nirje and Simon Olshansky et al., *The Principle of Normalization in Human Services* (Toronto, ON: National Institute on Mental Retardation, 1972), 28.
19. Perske, "The Dignity of Risk and the Mentally Retarded," 24.
20. Darold A. Treffert, "Dying with Their Rights On," *American Journal of* Psychiatry 130, no. 9 (September 1973): 1041.
21. Perske, "The Dignity of Risk and the Mentally Retarded," 24.
22. Treffert, "Dying with Their Rights On," 49.
23. United Nations Convention on the Rights of Persons with Disabilities (2006), Article 12, https://www.un.org/development/desa/disabilities/convention-on-the-rights-of-persons-with-disabilities/article-12-equal-recognition-before-the-law.html.
24. Fred Bayles, "Guardians of the Elderly: An Ailing System Part I: Declared 'Legally Dead' by a Troubled System," *Associated Press*, September 19, 1987, https://apnews.com/article/1198f64bb05d9c1ec690035983c02f9f.
25. Monthie, "The Myth of Liberty and Justice for All," 4.
26. Pamela B. Teaster, Erica F. Wood, Naomi Karp, et al., "Wards of the State: A National Study of Public Guardianship," The Retirement Research Foundation (2005), 3. https://www.americanbar.org/content/dam/aba/administrative/law_aging/wardofstatefinal.pdf
27. General Accounting Office, *Guardianships: Collaboration Needed to Protect Incapacitated Elderly People*, Publication Number GAO-04-655 (Washington, DC, 2004), 2.
28. Teaster et al., "Wards of the State," 4.
29. Carol D. Leonnig, Lena H. Sun, and Sarah Cohen, "Under Court, Vulnerable Became Victims," *Washington Post*, June 15, 2003. https://www.washingtonpost.com/archive/politics/2003/06/15/under-court-vulnerable-became-victims/859903d5-abc1-4751-8ae6-ab230b8a258e/.
30. Quoted in Teaster et al., "Wards of the State," 2.
31. Melvyn Colin Freeman, Kavitha Kolappy, Jose Miguel Caldas de Almeida, et al., "Reversing Hard Won Victories in the Name of Human Rights: A Critique of the General Comment on Article 12 of the UN Convention on the Rights of Persons with Disabilities," *Lancet Psychiatry* 2 (2015): 847–848.
32. United Nations Convention on the Rights of Persons with Disabilities, Article 12.
33. Gerard Quinn and Abigail Rekas-Rosalbo, "Civil Death: Rethinking the Foundations of Legal Personhood for Persons with a Disability," *Irish Jurist* 56 (2016): 289.
34. Freeman et al., "Reversing Hard Won Victories in the Name of Human Rights," 845.
35. Committee on the Rights of Persons with Disabilities, "General Comment No. 1" (2014), 1–2, https://www.ohchr.org/en/documents/general-comments-and-recommendations/general-comment-no-1-article-12-equal-recognition-1.
36. Freeman et al., "Reversing Hard Won Victories in the Name of Human Rights," 848.
37. Joseph Dute, "Should Substituted Decision-Making Be Abolished?" *European Journal of Health Law* 22 (2015): 318.
38. Law Society of Scotland, "Draft General Comment on Article 12 of the Convention—Equal Recognition Before the Law," November 2013, 5, 3. https://www.ohchr.org/_layouts/15/WopiFrame.aspx?sourcedoc=/Documents/HRBodies/CRPD/GC/LawSocietyOfScotlandArt12.doc&action=default&DefaultItemOpen=1.

39. Elizabeth Schroeder, "The Right to Decide: Developments in North American Guardianship Law," *GW Law International Law and Policy Brief*, March 21, 2022, https://studentbriefs.law.gwu.edu/ilpb/2022/03/21/the-right-to-decide-developments-in-north-american-guardianship-law-2/.
40. Quinn and Rekas-Rosalbo, "Civil Death," 312.
41. M. Browning, C. Bigby, and J. Douglas, "Supported Decision Making: Understanding How Its Conceptual Link to Legal Capacity Is Influencing the Development of Practice," *Research and Practice in Intellectual and Developmental Disabilities* 1 (2014): 36.
42. Autistic Self Advocacy Network, "The Right to Make Choices: International Laws and Decision-Making by People with Disabilities," 3, https://autisticadvocacy.org/wp-content/uploads/2016/02/Easy-Read-OSF-For-Families-v3.pdf.
43. Stephen Prutsman, Autism Society San Francisco Bay Area President, "SFASA Opposition to AB1663," March 7, 2022.
44. Jordan Page, "What the Free Britney Movement Did Next," *Vice*, January 20, 2022, https://www.vice.com/en/article/akv78a/when-did-the-free-britney-movement-end.
45. Gooding, *A New Era for Mental Health Law and Policy*, 243. For the lack of data on SDM, see also Karrie A. Shogren, Michael L. Wehmeyer, Heather Lassman, and Anjali J. Forber-Pratt, "Supported Decision Making," *Education and Training in Autism and Developmental Disabilities* 52, no. 2 (June 2017): 145, and N. A. Kohn, J. A. Blumenthal, and A. T. Campbell, "Supported Decision-Making: A Viable Alternative to Guardianship?," *Penn State Law Review* 117 (2013): 1128–1129.
46. Ronan Farrow and Jia Tolentino, "Britney Spears's Conservatorship Nightmare," *New Yorker*, July 3, 2021, https://www.newyorker.com/news/american-chronicles/britney-spears-conservatorship-nightmare?gclid=CjwKCAjwgISIBhBfEiwALE19SUbD-fCAwu4VEKMFofpzHmT48Na302Lv9nZnym-BCTNgmB4nGRAVoRoCuNcQAvD_BwE&source=google_sem_dom_promo.
47. Jill Escher, "Earth to Disability Activists: The Britney Spears Conservatorship Is Irrelevant to Cases of Adults with Severe Autism," National Council on Severe Autism Blog, July 28, 2021, https://www.ncsautism.org/blog//earth-to-disability-activists-the-britney-spears-conservatorship-is-irrelevant-to-cases-of-adults-with-severe-autism.
48. Reina Sultan, "The Horror of an Unwanted Conservatorship According to People Who Lived It," *Vice*, July 8, 2021, https://www.vice.com/en/article/epn57n/what-its-like-to-live-under-a-conservatorship-or-guardianship-britney-spears.
49. Escher, "Earth to Disability Activists."
50. "Rogers Guardianship," Mass.gov, https://www.mass.gov/rogers-guardianships.
51. Marina Sarris, "Antipsychotics and Autism: Weighing the Benefits, Eyeing the Risks," Interactive Autism Network, December 13, 2016, https://iancommunity.org/ssc/antipsychotics-and-autism-weighing-benefits-eyeing-risks.
52. Page, "What the Free Britney Movement Did Next."
53. John Elder Robison, "Does Mom Know Best, or Do We Presume Autistic Competence?," *Psychology Today*, January 22, 2016, https://www.psychologytoday.com/us/blog/my-life-aspergers/201601/does-mom-know-best-or-do-we-presume-autistic-competence.
54. Shogren et al., "Supported Decision Making," 149.
55. Hannah Brown, "Take the Autism Challenge," *Huffington Post*, March 30, 2017, https://www.huffpost.com/entry/please-run-on-april-2-for-world-autism-awareness-day_b_58dcacbee4b04ba4a5e250de.
56. John Elder Robison and Amy Lutz transcript, March 8, 2019.

Chapter 6

1. Peyton Goddard and Dianne Goddard, with Carol Cujec, *I Am Intelligent: From Heartbreak to Healing—A Mother and Daughter's Journey through Autism* (Guilford, CT: skirt!, 2012), 173.
2. Douglas Biklen, Mary Winston Morton, and Deborah Gold et al., "Facilitated Communication: Implications for Individuals with Autism," *Topics in Language Disorders* 12 (August 1992): 5.
3. Jon Palfreman, "The Australian Origins of Facilitated Communication," in *Facilitated Communication: The Clinical and Social Phenomenon*, Howard Shane, ed. (San Diego, CA: Singular, 1994), 54.
4. Laura Schreibman, *The Science and Fiction of Autism* (Cambridge, MA: Harvard University Press, 2005), 204.
5. Howard C. Shane, "Facilitated Communication: Factual, Fictional, or Factitious," in *Facilitated Communication*, 3.
6. Diane Twachtman-Cullen, *A Passion to Believe: Autism and the Facilitated Communication Phenomenon* (Boulder, CO: Westview Press, 1997), 11.
7. Douglas Biklen, "Communication Unbound: Autism and Praxis," *Harvard Educational Review* 60, no. 3 (August 1990): 312.
8. Scott O. Lilienfeld, Julia Marshall, and James T. Todd et al., "The Persistence of Fad Interventions in the Face of Negative Scientific Evidence: Facilitated Communication for Autism as a Case Example," *Evidence-Based Communication Assessment and Intervention* (2015): 67.
9. Gina Green, "Facilitated Communication: Mental Miracle or Sleight of Hand?" *Behavior and Social Issues* 4, no. 1–2 (1994): 80.
10. Kenneth N. Margolin, "How Shall Facilitated Communication Be Judged? Facilitated Communication and the Legal System," in *Facilitated Communication*, 239.
11. Lilienfeld et al., "The Persistence of Fad Interventions," 70.
12. Ralf W. Schlosser, Susan Balandin, Bronwyn Hemsley, et al., "Facilitated Communication and Authorship: A Systematic Review," *Augmentative and Alternative Communication* 30, no. 4 (2014): 359; Bronwyn Hemsley, Lucy Bryant, Ralf W. Schlosser, et al., "Systematic Review of Facilitated Communication 2014–2018 Finds No New Evidence That Messages Delivered Using Facilitated Communication Are Authored by the Person with Disability," *Autism & Developmental Language Impairments* 3 (2018): 1–8.
13. William Paul Simmons, Janyce Boynton, and Todd Landman, "Facilitated Communication, Neurodiversity, and Human Rights," *Human Rights Quarterly* 43, no. 1 (February 2021): 155.
14. Ashli A. Owen-Smith, Stephen Bent, Frances L. Lynch, et al., "Prevalence and Predictors of Complementary and Alternative Medicine Use in a Large Insured Sample of Children with Autism Spectrum Disorders," *Research in Autism Spectrum Disorders* 17 (September 2015): 40.
15. Daniel Engber, "The Strange Case of Anna Stubblefield," *New York Times Magazine*, October 20, 2015, https://www.New Yorktimes.com/2015/10/25/magazine/the-strange-case-of-anna-stubblefield.html. Stubblefield's conviction was overturned in 2017 because the Appellate Court determined that Rosemary Crossley, one of the earliest practitioners of FC, had been wrongfully prohibited from testifying for the defense. Stubblefield pled guilty to a lesser charge of aggravated criminal sexual contact and was sentenced to time served.

16. J. B. Handley and Jamison Handley, *Underestimated: An Autism Miracle* (New York: Skyhorse, 2021), 139.
17. Brendan Borrell, "How One Communication Tool May Fail Some Autistic People," *Spectrum*, July 1, 2020, https://www.spectrumnews.org/features/deep-dive/how-one-communication-tool-may-fail-some-autistic-people/.
18. Iversen, *Strange Son*, 74.
19. Goddard and Goddard, *I Am Intelligent*, 1.
20. Handley and Handley, *Underestimated*, 6.
21. Gilpeer and Grodin, *I Have Been Buried under Years of Dust*, 4.
22. Matthew Hobson and Nancy Hobson, *I'm So Glad You Found Me in Here* (New York: Ithaca Press, 2010).
23. Goddard and Goddard, *I am Intelligent*, 53, 26.
24. Levin, *Unlocked*, 101.
25. Barron and Barron, *There's a Boy in Here*, 232.
26. Stacey, *The Boy Who Loved Windows*, 232.
27. McCarthy, *Louder than Words*, 186.
28. Savarese, *Reasonable People*, 407, 411.
29. Elizabeth M. Bonker and Virginia G. Breen, *I Am in Here: The Journey of a Child with Autism Who Cannot Speak but Finds Her Voice* (Grand Rapids, MI: Revell, 2011), 228.
30. Goddard and Goddard, *I Am Intelligent*, 208.
31. Russell Martin, *Out of Silence: A Journey into Language* (New York: Henry Holt, 1994), 233.
32. Ibid., 222.
33. Savarese, *Reasonable People*, xv.
34. Naoki Higashida, *The Reason I Jump* (New York: Random House, 2013), 21.
35. Gilpeer and Grodin, *I Have Been Buried under Years of Dust*, 199.
36. Twachtman-Cullen, *A Passion to Believe*, 5.
37. Karen Chenausky, Amanda Brignell, Angela Morgan, and Helen Tager-Flusberg, "Motor Speech Impairment Predicts Expressive Language in Minimally Verbal, but Not Low Verbal, Individuals with Autism Spectrum Disorder," *Autism & Developmental Language Impairments* 4 (2019): 2; 1–12.
38. Shane, "Facilitated Communication: Factual, Fictional, or Factitious," 11.
39. Gilpeer and Grodin, *I Have Been Buried under Years of Dust*, 120, 134.
40. Handley and Handley, *Underestimated*, 94.
41. Goddard and Goddard, *I Am Intelligent*, 69.
42. Ido Kedar, *Ido in Autismland: Climbing Out of Autism's Silent Prison* (self-published, 2012), 45.
43. Goddard and Goddard, *I Am Intelligent*, 208.
44. Gilpeer and Grodin, *I Have Been Buried under Years of Dust*, 92.
45. Kedar, *Ido in Autismland*, 27.
46. Kedar, *Ido in Autismland*, 71–72.
47. Shane, "Facilitated Communication: Factual, Fictional, or Factitious," 13.
48. Marianne Leone, *Jesse: A Mother's Story* (New York: Simon & Schuster, 2010), 37.
49. John W. Jacobson, James A. Mulick, and Allen A. Schwartz, "A History of Facilitated Communication: Science, Pseudoscience, and Antiscience Working Group on Facilitated Communication," *American Psychologist* 50, no. 9 (1995): 755.
50. Michael Rutter, "Concepts of Autism: A Review of Research," *Journal of Child Psychology and Psychiatry* 9 (1968): 15, 17.

51. Ibid., 18.
52. Wing, "Asperger's Syndrome," 117.
53. Nancy J. Minshew, Gerald Goldstein, and Don J. Siegel, "Speech and Language in High-Functioning Autistic Individuals," *Neuropsychology* 9, no. 2 (1995): 258. See also Gabriella Rundblad and Dagmara Annaz, "The Atypical Development of Metaphor and Metonymy Comprehension in Children with Autism," *Autism: The International Journal of Research and Practice* 14, no. 1 (2010): 40.
54. Francesca G. E. Happé, "Understanding Minds and Metaphors: Insights from the Study of Figurative Language in Autism," *Metaphor and Symbolic Activity* 10, no. 4 (1995): 276.
55. R. Peter Hobson and Anthony Lee, "Emotion-Related and Abstract Concepts in Autistic People: Evidence from the British Picture Vocabulary Scale," *Journal of Autism and Developmental Disorders* 19 (1989): 601.
56. Helen Tager-Flusberg, "Autistic Children's Talk about Psychological States: Deficits in the Early Acquisition of a Theory of Mind," *Child Development* 63 (1992): 161.
57. So Hyun Kim, Rhea Paul, Helen Tager-Flusberg, and Catherine Lord, "Language and Communication in Autism," in *Handbook of Autism and Pervasive Developmental Disorders*, Vol. 1: *Diagnosis, Development, and Brain Mechanisms*, 4th edition, Fred R. Volkmar, Sally J. Rogers, Reha Paul, and Kevin A. Pelphrey, eds. (Hoboken, NJ: John Wiley & Sons, 2014), 250.
58. Minshew, Goldstein, and Siegel, "Speech and Language in High-Functioning Autistic Individuals," 258.
59. Martin, *Out of Silence*, 264.
60. Hobson and Hobson, *I'm So Glad You Found Me in Here*, 60, 62.
61. Savarese, *Reasonable People*, 138.
62. Handley and Handley, *Underestimated*, 91, 116.
63. Evon Z. Vogt and Ray Hyman, *Water Witching U.S.A.* (Chicago: University of Chicago Press, 1959), 132, 119.
64. Douglas Keith Candland, *Feral Children and Clever Animals: Reflections on Human Nature* (New York: Oxford University Press, 1993), 118, 169.
65. Wolf Wolfensberger, "The 'Facilitated Communication' Craze as an Instance of Pathological Science: The Cold Fusion of Human Services," in *Facilitated Communication*, 87.
66. Shane, "The Facilitated Nightmare: The Dark Side of the Phenomenon," in *Facilitated Communication*, 315.
67. John V. Petrocelli, *The Life-Changing Science of Detecting Bullshit* (New York: St. Martin's Press, 2021), 260, 262.
68. Simmons, Boynton, and Landsman, "Facilitated Communication, Neurodiversity, and Human Rights," 157.
69. Hobson, *I'm So Glad You Found Me in Here*, 59.
70. Handley and Handley, *Underestimated*, 86.
71. Biklen, "Communication Unbound," 310.
72. Savarese, *Reasonable People*, xxii.
73. Handley, *Underestimated*, 141.
74. Biklen, "Communication Unbound," 310.
75. Kedar, *Ido in Autismland*, 98.
76. Iversen, *Strange Son*, 119.
77. Ibid., 248–249.

78. David Jaher, *The Witch of Lime Street: Séance, Seduction, and Houdini in the Spirit World* (New York: Broadway Books, 2015).
79. Vogt and Hyman, *Water Witching U.S.A.*, 118.
80. Handley and Handley, *Underestimated*, 86.
81. Martin, *Out of Silence*, 232.
82. Howard C. Shane, "Establishing the Source of Communication," in *Facilitated Communication*, 292.
83. Martin, *Out of Silence*, 205, 286.
84. Jennifer Binder Le-Pape, "An Open Letter to My Son's Skeptics," I-ASC, March 3, 2021, https://i-asc.org/an-open-letter-to-my-sons-skeptics/.
85. Gina Green, "The Quality of the Evidence," in *Facilitated Communication*, 168.
86. Green, "Facilitated Communication," 77.
87. Michael J. Salomon Weiss and Sheldon H. Wagner, "Emerging Validation of Facilitated Communication: New Findings about Old Assumptions," in *Contested Words, Contested Science: Unraveling the Facilitated Communication Controversy*, Douglas Biklen and Donald N. Cardinal, eds. (New York: Teachers College Press, 1997), 155.
88. Biklen, "Communication Unbound," 307.
89. Douglas Biklen and Donald N. Cardinal, "Framing the Issue: Author or Not, Competent or Not?" in *Contested Words, Contested Science*, 32.
90. HALO (Helping Autism through Learning and Outreach), "Scientific Research into Soma RPM," https://www.halo-soma.org/research.
91. Jacobson, Mulick, and Schwartz, "A History of Facilitated Communication," 756.
92. Gregory C. Tino, *The Autistic Mind Finally Speaks: Letterboard Thoughts* (Independently published, 2020), 45.
93. National Institute for Health and Care Excellence, "Autism Spectrum Disorder in Under 19s: Support and Management," June 14, 2021, https://pubmed.ncbi.nlm.nih.gov/34283415/.
94. Green, "The Quality of the Evidence," 215.
95. Paul Haskew and Anne Donnellan, *Emotional Maturity and Well-Being: Psychological Lessons of Facilitated Communication* (Madison, WI: DRI Press, 1993), 9.
96. Jennifer Binder Le-Pape, "An Open Letter to My Son's Skeptics."
97. Vikram K. Jaswal, Allison Wayne, and Hudson Golino, "Eye-Tracking Reveals Agency in Assisted Autistic Communication," *Scientific Reports* 10 (2020): 7882, https://www.nature.com/articles/s41598-020-64553-9. This study has received the most attention by far of these three; for critiques, see Katherine Beals, "A Recent Eye-Tracking Study Fails to Reveal Agency in Assisted Autistic Communication," *Evidence-Based Communication Assessment and Intervention* 15, no. 1 (2021): 46–51, and Stuart Vyse, "Of Eye Movements and Autism: The Latest Chapter in a Continuing Controversy," *Skeptical Inquirer* (May 30, 2020), https://skepticalinquirer.org/exclusive/of-eye-movements-and-autism-the-latest-chapter-in-a-continuing-controversy/.
98. I-ASC, "Studying Receptive Language in Nonspeakers through Brain Imaging," https://i-asc.org/wp-content/uploads/2020/06/2-STUDYING-RECEPTIVE-LANGUAGE-IN-NONSPEAKERS-THROUGH-BRAIN-IMAGING.pdf.
99. Patrick Faure, Thierry Legou, and Bruno Gepner, "Evidence of Authorship on Messages in Facilitated Communication: A Case Report Using Accelerometry," *Frontiers in Psychiatry* 11 (December 2020).
100. Bonker and Breen, *I Am in Here*, 223.

101. Tino, *The Autistic Mind Finally Speaks*, 31, 46.
102. Simmons, Boynton, and Landman, "Facilitated Communication, Neurodiversity, and Human Rights," 148.
103. Wolfensberger, "The 'Facilitated Communication' Craze as an Instance of Pathological Science," 63. The term "pathological science" is credited to Nobel Prize–winning chemist Irving Langmuir, who defined it as "the science of things that aren't so."
104. Kathy Sundstrom, "Carer: 'I Fell in Love': Grandma Guilty of Indecent Dealing," *Sunshine Coast Daily*, October 16, 2014, www.couriermail.com.au%2Fnews%2Fqueensland%2Fsunshine-coast%2Fi-love-him-disability-carer-faces-court-over-love-affair%2Fnews-.story%2F17d74d010a2f3d266a4143047810484a&usg=AOvVaw2aTjTJBqm0rlDtbh5Y_xnE.
105. Sarah Kaplan, "The Millionaire Mom Who Poisoned Her Autistic Son and Called It a Mercy Killing," *Washington Post*, May 29, 2015, https://www.washingtonpost.com/news/morning-mix/wp/2015/05/29/a-murder-or-a-mercy-killing-the-tangled-and-troubling-trial-of-gigi-jordan/.
106. Gretchen Scheibel, Thomas L. Zane, and Kathleen N. Zimmerman, "An Economic Evaluation of Emerging and Ineffective Interventions: Examining the Role of Cost When Translating Research into Practice," *Exceptional Children* 88, no. 3 (January 20, 2022): 245..
107. Kedar, *Ido in Autismland*, 56.
108. Kathleen M. Dillon, "Facilitated Communication, Autism, and Ouija," *The Skeptical Inquirer* 17, no. 3 (1993): 285.
109. Barry M. Prizant, Amy M. Wetherby, and Patrick J. Rydell, "Implications of Facilitated Communication for Education and Communication Enhancement Practices for Persons with Autism," in *Facilitated Communication*, 138, 143.
110. Savarese, *Reasonable People*, 192, 195.
111. Higashida, *The Reason I Jump*, 86.
112. Kedar, *Ido in Autismland*, 53.
113. Martin, *Out of Silence*, 238.
114. Tino, *The Autistic Mind Finally Speaks*, 50–51.
115. United for Communication Choice press release, July 2018, https://unitedforcommunicationchoice.org/national-coalition-opposes-ashas-attempts-to-restrict-communication-choice/950/.
116. Jeffrey Chan and Karen Nankervis, "Stolen Voices: Facilitated Communication Is an Abuse of Human Rights," *Evidence-Based Communication Assessment and Intervention* 8, no. 3 (2014): 151–153.
117. United Nations, *Convention on the Rights of Persons with Disabilities* (2006), https://www.un.org/development/desa/disabilities/convention-on-the-rights-of-persons-with-disabilities.html.
118. Jennifer B. Ganz, Anonis Katsiyannis, and Kristi L. Morin, "Facilitated Communication: The Resurgence of a Disproven Treatment for Individuals with Autism," *Intervention in School and Clinic* 54, no. 1 (2018): 52, 54.
119. Victoria F. Knight, Heartley B. Huber, Emily M. Kuntz, et al., "Instructional Practices, Priorities, and Preparedness for Educating Students with Autism and Intellectual Disability," *Focus on Autism and Other Developmental Disabilities* 34, no. 1 (March 2019): 13.

120. Bill Chappell, "A Nonspeaking Valedictorian with Autism Gives Her College's Commencement Speech," *NPR*, May 12, 2022, https://www.npr.org/2022/05/12/1098506522/nonspeaking-valedictorian-autism-college-commencement-speech.
121. Martin Gardner, "Facilitated Communication: A Cruel Farce," *Skeptical Inquirer* 25, no. 1 (January–February 2001), 18.
122. Lyanne Melendez, "2 UC Berkeley Students Make History as 1st Nonspeaking Autistic Graduates," *ABC 7 News*, May 19, 2022, https://abc7news.com/uc-berkeley-cal-graduation-nonspeaking-autism-graduates-david-teplitz/11870714/.
123. James T. Todd, "The Moral Obligation to Be Empirical: Comments on Boynton's 'Facilitated Communication—What Harm Can It Do: Confessions of a Former Facilitator,'" *Evidence-Based Communication Assessment and Intervention* (2012): 1–22.
124. Handley and Handley, *Underestimated*, 34.
125. Kedar, *Ido in Autismland*, 54.
126. Bonker and Breen, *I Am in Here*, 213.
127. Kedar, *Ido in Autismland*, 36.
128. Bonker and Breen, *I Am in Here*, 81.
129. Goddard and Goddard, *I Am Intelligent*, 16.
130. Savarese, *Reasonable People*, 333.
131. Tino, *The Autistic Mind Finally Speaks*, 52.
132. Handley, *Underestimated*, 155.
133. See Kedar, *Ido in Autismland*, 134; Gilpeer and Grodin, *I Have Been Buried under Years of Dust*, 241; Goddard and Goddard, *I Am Intelligent*, 269.
134. Bonker and Breen, *I Am in Here*, 130.
135. Higashida, *The Reason I Jump*, xvi.
136. Gilpeer and Grodin, *I Have Been Buried under Years of Dust*, 198.
137. Iversen, *Strange Son*, 370.
138. Kedar, *Ido in Autismland*, 76.

Conclusion

1. Katie O'Neill and Rebecca McCarthy, "The Pitfalls of Presumptions," *The ASHA Leader*, December 1, 2018, https://leader.pubs.asha.org/doi/10.1044/leader.FMP.23122018.10.
2. Jason Travers and Kevin M. Ayres, "A Critique of Presuming Competence of Learners with Autism or Other Developmental Disabilities," *Education and Training in Autism and Developmental Disabilities* 50, no. 4 (December 2015): 372.
3. Anne M. Donnellan, "The Criterion of the Least Dangerous Assumption," *Behavioral Disorders* 9, no. 2 (February 1984): 142; 141–150.
4. Handley, *Underestimated*, 155.
5. Borrell, "How One Communication Tool May Fail Some Autistic People."
6. Christopher Kliewer, Douglas Biklen, and Amy J. Petersen, "At the End of Intellectual Disability," *Harvard Educational Review* 85, no. 1 (Spring 2015): 22; 1–28..
7. Davis, *Breaking Autism's Barriers*, 33.
8. Robert Hughes, *Walker Finds a Way: Running into the Adult World with Autism* (London: Jessica Kingsley, 2016), 45.
9. Greenfeld, *A Place for Noah*, 48.

10. Amy S. F. Lutz, "Baseline," in Lutz, *We Walk: Life with Severe Autism* (Ithaca, NY: Cornell University Press, 2020), 140.
11. Travers and Ayres, "A Critique of Presuming Competence of Learners with Autism or Other Developmental Disabilities," 373, 377, 379, 375, 377.
12. Carol Gilligan, *In a Different Voice: Psychological Theory and Women's Development* (Cambridge, MA: Harvard University Press, 1982), 74.
13. Joan C. Tronto, *Moral Boundaries: A Political Argument for an Ethic of Care* (New York: Routledge, 1993), 119.
14. Kittay, *Learning from My Daughter*, 167.
15. Arthur Kleinman, *The Soul of Care: The Moral Education of a Husband and a Doctor* (New York: Viking, 2019), 128, 245.
16. Kittay, *Learning from My Daughter*, xx.
17. Tronto, *Moral Boundaries*, 145.
18. Tronto, *Moral Boundaries*, 145.
19. Kittay, *Learning from My Daughter*, 174.
20. Lisa Freitag, *Extreme Caregiving: The Moral Work of Raising Children with Special Needs* (New York: Oxford University Press, 2018), 62.
21. Allison C. Carey, Pamela Block, and Richard K. Scotch, *Allies and Obstacles: Disability Activism and Parents of Children with Disabilities* (Philadelphia: Temple University Press, 2020).
22. Abby Maslin, *Love You Hard: A Memoir of Marriage, Brain Injury, and Reinventing Love* (New York: Dutton, 2019), 97.
23. Kate Washington, *Already Toast: Caregiving and Burnout in America* (Boston: Beacon Press, 2021), 31.
24. Cynthia Lim, *Wherever You Are: A Memoir of Love, Marriage, and Brain Injury* (Kenmore, WA: Coffeetown Press, 2018), 70–71.
25. Maslin, *Love You Hard*, 165.
26. Tronto, *Moral Boundaries*, 136.
27. Eva Feder Kittay, *Love's Labor: Essays on Women, Equality, and Dependency* (New York: Routledge, 1999), 143.
28. The National Alliance for Caregiving and AARP, "Caregiving in the U.S. 2020," https://www.caregiving.org/caregiving-in-the-us-2020/.
29. Tronto, *Moral Boundaries*, 105.
30. Kittay, *Learning from My Daughter*, 175, 191.
31. Autistic Self-Advocacy Network, "Keeping the Promise: Self Advocates Defining the Meaning of Community Living," pp. 6–7, https://autisticadvocacy.org/wp-content/uploads/2012/02/KeepingthePromise-SelfAdvocatesDefiningtheMeaningofCommunity.pdf.
32. Ari Ne'eman, "Watch the Appointments," *Sometimes a Lion*, January 21, 2017, https://arineeman.com/2017/01/22/watch-the-appointments/.
33. Amy S. F. Lutz, "Ideology, Not Data," *Psychology Today*, January 22, 2017, https://www.psychologytoday.com/us/blog/inspectrum/201701/ideology-not-data.
34. David S. Mandell, "A House Is Not a Home: The Great Residential Divide in Autism Care," *Autism*, September 10, 2017, https://journals.sagepub.com/doi/full/10.1177/1362361317722101.
35. Amy S. F. Lutz, "The Reverse Field of Dreams Fallacy in Disability Policy," *Psychology Today*, November 8, 2021, https://www.psychologytoday.com/us/blog/inspectrum/202111/the-reverse-field-dreams-fallacy-in-disability-policy.

36. Christina Jewett, "Nowhere to Go: Young People with Autism Languish in Hospitals," *Kaiser Health News*, September 26, 2017, https://khn.org/news/for-thousands-of-autistic-teens-hospital-ers-serve-as-home/.
37. Jason Laughlin, "Nowhere to Go," *Philadelphia Inquirer*, November 5, 2021, https://www.inquirer.com/health/a/autism-treatment-therapy-care-hospital-health-system-20211105.html.
38. Karl Taro Greenfeld, *Boy Alone: A Brother's Memoir* (New York: Harper Perennial, 2009), 174.
39. Ibid., 283.
40. Ibid., 329–330.
41. Ibid., 329.

Bibliography

Anderson, Connie, J. Kiely Law, Amy Daniels, et al. "Occurrence and Family Impact of Elopement in Children with Autism Spectrum Disorders." *Pediatrics* 130, no. 5 (November 1, 2012): 870–877.

Anderson, Deborah K., Jessie W. Liang, and Catherine Lord. "Predicting Young Adult Outcome among More and Less Cognitively Able Individuals with Autism Spectrum Disorders." *The Journal of Child Psychology and Psychiatry* 55, no. 5 (2014): 485–494.

Apgar, Amanda. *The Disabled Child: Memoirs of a Normal Future*. Ann Arbor: University of Michigan Press, 2023.

Appelbaum, Paul S. "There Are All Kinds of Rights." *The Hastings Center Report* 46, no. 2 (March–April 2016): inside back cover.

Autistic Self-Advocacy Network. "About ASAN." https://autisticadvocacy.org/about-asan/.

Autistic Self-Advocacy Network. "The Right to Make Choices: International Laws and Decision-Making by People with Disabilities." 2016. https://autisticadvocacy.org/wp-content/uploads/2016/02/Easy-Read-OSF-For-Families-v3.pdf.

Autistic Self-Advocacy Network, Self Advocates Becoming Empowered, and the National Youth Leadership Network. "Keeping the Promise: Self Advocates Defining the Meaning of Community Living." 2012. https://autisticadvocacy.org/wp-content/uploads/2012/02/KeepingthePromise-SelfAdvocatesDefiningtheMeaningofCommunity.pdf

Axline, Virginia M. *Dibs in Search of Self*. New York: Ballantine Books, 1964.

Baker, Anthony D. "Recognizing Jake: Contending with Formulaic and Spectacularized Representations of Autism in Film." In *Autism and Representation*, edited by Mark Osteen, 229–243. New York: Routledge, 2008.

Baldwin, Alfred L. "Current Trends of Research in Child Development." In *Psychopathology of Childhood*, edited by Paul H. Hoch and Joseph Zubin, 25–31. New York: Grune and Stratton, 1955.

Barker, John Wayne. "Sameness." Bark's Bytes, Blog of Merrick, Inc. (November 9, 2021). https://merrickinc.org/barks-bytes/barks-bytes-43-sameness/.

Barron, Judy, and Sean Barron. *There's a Boy in Here: A Mother and Her Son Tell the Story of His Emergence from Autism*. Arlington, TX: Future Horizons, 2002.

Barry, Dan. "The 'Boys' in the Bunkhouse: Toil, Abuse and Endurance in the Heartland." *New York Times*, March 9, 2014. https://www.New Yorktimes.com/interactive/2014/03/09/us/the-boys-in-the-bunkhouse.html.

Bayles, Fred. "Guardians of the Elderly: An Ailing System Part I: Declared 'Legally Dead' by a Troubled System." *Associated Press*, September 19, 1987. https://apnews.com/article/1198f64bb05d9c1ec690035983c02f9f.

Beals, Katherine. "A Recent Eye-Tracking Study Fails to Reveal Agency in Assisted Autistic Communication." *Evidence-Based Communication Assessment and Intervention* 15, no. 1 (2021): 46–51.

Beck, Martha. *Expecting Adam: A True Story of Birth, Rebirth, and Everyday Magic*. New York: Three Rivers Press, 1999.

Benda, Clemens E. *The Child with Mongolism (Congenital Acromicria)*. New York: Grune and Stratton, 1960.

Benda, Clemens E. *Developmental Disorders of Mentation and Cerebral Palsies*. New York: Grune & Stratton, 1952.

Bender, Lauretta. "Autism in Children with Mental Deficiency." *American Journal of Mental Deficiency* 64, no. 1 (January 1959): 81–86.

Bender, Lauretta. "The Development of a Schizophrenic Child Treated with Electric Convulsions at Three Years of Age." In *Emotional Problems of Early Childhood*, edited by Gerald Caplan, 407–425. New York: Basic Books, 1955.

Bender, Lauretta. *Psychopathology of Children with Organic Brain Disorders*. Springfield, IL: Charles C. Thomas, 1956.

Bettelheim, Bruno. *The Empty Fortress: Infantile Autism and the Birth of the Self*. New York: Free Press, 1967.

Bickel, Horst. John Gerrard, and Evelyn M. Hickmans. "The Influence of Phenylalanine Intake on the Chemistry and Behaviour of a Phenylketonuric Child." *Acta Paediatrica* 43 (January 1954): 64–77.

Biklen, Douglas. "Communication Unbound: Autism and Praxis." *Harvard Educational Review* 60, no. 3 (August 1990): 291–315.

Biklen, Douglas, and Donald N. Cardinal. "Framing the Issue: Author or Not, Competent or Not?" In *Contested Words, Contested Science: Unraveling the Facilitated Communication Controversy*, edited by Douglas Biklen and Donald N. Cardinal, 5–33. New York: Teachers College Press, 1997.

Biklen, Douglas, Mary Winston Morton, and Deborah Gold. "Facilitated Communication: Implications for Individuals with Autism." *Topics in Language Disorders* 12 (August 1992): 1–28.

Blum, Deborah. *Love at Goon Park*. Cambridge, MA: Perseus, 2002.

Bonker, Elizabeth M., and Virginia G. Breen. *I Am in Here: The Journey of a Child with Autism Who Cannot Speak but Finds Her Voice*. Grand Rapids, MI: Revell, 2011.

Borrell, Brendan. "How One Communication Tool May Fail Some Autistic People." *Spectrum*, July 1, 2020. https://www.spectrumnews.org/features/deep-dive/how-one-communication-tool-may-fail-some-autistic-people/.

Bottema-Beutel, Kristen, Steven K. Kapp, Jessica Nina Lester, et al. "Avoiding Ableist Language: Suggestions for Autism Researchers." *Autism in Adulthood* 3, no. 1 (2021): 18–29. https://www-liebertpub-com.proxy.library.upenn.edu/doi/epdf/10.1089/aut.2020.0014.

Bowlby, John. *Maternal Care and Mental Health: A Report Prepared on Behalf of the World Health Organization as a Contribution to the United Nations Programme for the Welfare of Homeless Children*. Geneva: World Health Organization, 1951.

Bowlby, John. *Attachment and Loss*, Vol. I: *Attachment*. New York: Basic Books, 1969.

Branson, Jan, and Don Miller. "Sign Language, the Deaf and the Epistemic Violence of Mainstreaming." *Language and Education* 7, no. 1 (1993): 21–41.

Brousseau, Kate. *Mongolism: A Study of the Physical and Mental Characteristics of Mongolian Imbeciles*. Baltimore, MD: Williams & Wilkins, 1928.

Brown, Christy. *My Left Foot*. London: Secker and Warburg, 1954.

Brown, Hannah. "Take the Autism Challenge." *Huffington Post*, March 30, 2017. https://www.huffpost.com/entry/please-run-on-april-2-for-world-autism-awareness-day_b_58dcacbee4b04ba4a5e250de

Brown, Helene. *Yesterday's Child*. New York: Signet, 1977.

Brown, Ian. *The Boy in the Moon*. New York: St. Martin's Press, 2009.

Browning, M., C. Bigby, and J. Douglas. "Supported Decision Making: Understanding How Its Conceptual Link to Legal Capacity Is Influencing the Development of Practice." *Research and Practice in Intellectual and Developmental Disabilities* 1 (2014): 34–45.

Buck, Pearl S. *The Child Who Never Grew*. New York: John Day, 1950.

Buck, Pearl S. *The Gifts They Bring: Our Debt to the Mentally Retarded*. New York: John Day, 1965.

Buhrer, Eliza. "Mental Competency Inquisitions from Medieval England (ca. late 12th c.–early 15th c.)." In *Medieval Disability Sourcebook*, edited by Cameron Hunt McNabb, 56–68. Santa Barbara, CA: Punctum Books, 2020.

Burghardt, Madeline C. *Broken: Institutions, Families, and the Construction of Intellectual Disability*. Montreal: McGill-Queen's University Press, 2018.

Candland, Douglas Keith. *Feral Children and Clever Animals: Reflections on Human Nature*. New York: Oxford University Press, 1995.

Carey, Allison C. "Parents and Professionals: Parents' Reflections on Professionals, the Support System, and the Family in the Twentieth-Century United States." In *Disability Histories*, edited by Susan Burch and Michael Rembis, 58–76. Springfield: University of Illinois Press, 2014.

Carey, Allison C., Pamela Block, and Richard K. Scotch. *Allies and Obstacles: Disability Activism and Parents of Children with Disabilities*. Philadelphia: Temple University Press, 2020.

Carlson, Earl R. *Born That Way*. New York: John Day, 1941.

Castles, Katherine. "'Nice, Average Americans': Postwar Parents' Groups and the Defense of the Normal Family." In *Mental Retardation in America: A Historical Reader*, edited by Steven Noll and James W. Trent, Jr., 351–370. New York: New York University Press, 2004.

Center for Health Care Strategies. "Trends and Challenges in Publicly-Financed Care for Individuals with Intellectual and Developmental Disabilities." September 2012. http://www.chcs.org/media/IDD_Service_Delivery_Systems_082812.pdf.

Center for Public Representation. "U.S. Supported Decision-Making Laws." 2023. https://supporteddecisions.org/resources-on-sdm/state-supported-decision-making-laws-and-court-decisions/.

Centers for Disease Control and Prevention. "Facts about Developmental Disabilities." 2022. https://www.cdc.gov/ncbddd/developmentaldisabilities/facts.html.

Chan, Jeffrey, and Karen Nankervis. "Stolen Voices: Facilitated Communication Is an Abuse of Human Rights." *Evidence-Based Communication Assessment and Intervention* 8, no. 3 (2014): 151–156.

Chappell, Bill. "A Nonspeaking Valedictorian with Autism Gives Her College's Commencement Speech." *NPR*, May 12, 2022. https://www.npr.org/2022/05/12/1098506522/nonspeaking-valedictorian-autism-college-commencement-speech.

Chenausky, Karen, Amanda Brignell, Angela Morgan, and Helen Tager-Flusberg. "Motor Speech Impairment Predicts Expressive Language in Minimally Verbal, but Not Low Verbal, Individuals with Autism Spectrum Disorder." *Autism & Developmental Language Impairments* 4 (2019): 1–12.

Committee on the Rights of Persons with Disabilities. "General Comment No. 1." 2014. https://www.ohchr.org/en/documents/general-comments-and-recommendations/general-comment-no-1-article-12-equal-recognition-1.

Copeland, James, with Jack Hodges. *For the Love of Ann*. New York: Ballantine Books, 1973.

Costandi, Moheb. "Against Neurodiversity." *Aeon*, September 12, 2019. https://aeon.co/essays/why-the-neurodiversity-movement-has-become-harmful.

Couser, G. Thomas. *Signifying Bodies: Disability in Contemporary Life Writing*. Ann Arbor: University of Michigan Press, 2009.

Couser, G. Thomas. "Introduction: Disability and Life Writing." *Journal of Literary & Cultural Disability Studies* 5, no. 3 (2011): 229–242.

Crocker, A. G., C. Mercier, and Y. Lachapelle. "Prevalence and Types of Aggressive Behaviour among Adults with Intellectual Disabilities." *Journal of Intellectual Disability Research* 50 (September 2006): 652–661.

Davis, Bill. *Breaking Autism's Barriers: A Father's Story*. London: Jessica Kingsley, 2001.

Davis, Lennard J. *Enabling Acts: The Hidden Story of How the Americans with Disabilities Act Gave the Largest US Minority Its Rights*. Boston: Beacon Press, 2016.

Deacon, Joseph John. *Joey: An Unforgettable Story of Human Courage*. New York: Charles Scribner's Sons, 1974.

Decoteau, Claire Laurier, and Meghan Daniel. "Scientific Hegemony and the Field of Autism." *American Sociological Review* 85, no. 3 (June 2020): 1–26.

DeMyer, Marian K. *Parents and Children in Autism*. New York: John Wiley & Sons, 1979.

Despert, J. Louise. *The Emotionally Disturbed Child: Then and Now*. New York: Robert Brunner, 1965.

Dillon, Kathleen M. "Facilitated Communication, Autism, and Ouija." *Skeptical Inquirer* 17, no. 3 (1993): 281–287.

Dinerstein, Robert. "Implementing Legal Capacity under Article 12 of the UN Convention on the Rights of Persons with Disabilities: The Difficult Road from Guardianship to Supported Decision Making." *Human Rights Brief* 19, no. 2 (2012): 8–9.

Dolnick, Edward. *Madness on the Couch: Blaming the Victim in the Heyday of Psychoanalysis*. New York: Simon & Schuster, 1998.

Donnellan, Anne M. "The Criterion of the Least Dangerous Assumption." *Behavioral Disorders* 9, no. 2 (February 1984): 141–150.

Donvan, John, and Caren Zucker. *In a Different Key: The Story of Autism*. New York: Crown, 2016.

Dugdale, Richard L. *The Jukes: A Study in Crime, Pauperism, Disease and Heredity*. New York: G. P. Putnam's Sons, 1877.

Dute, Joseph. "Should Substituted Decision-Making Be Abolished?" *European Journal of Health Law* 22 (2015): 315–320.

Dwyer, Patrick, Jacalyn G. Ryan, Zachary J. Williams, and Dena L. Gassner. "First Do No Harm: Suggestions Regarding Respectful Autism Language." *Pediatrics* 149, no. s4 (April 2022): 1–3. https://publications-aap-org.proxy.library.upenn.edu/pediatrics/article/149/Supplement%204/e2020049437N/185653/First-Do-No-Harm-Suggestions-Regarding-Respectful?autologincheck=redirected

Edgerton, Robert B. *The Cloak of Competence: Stigma in the Lives of the Mentally Retarded*. Berkeley: University of California Press, 1967.

Ehrenreich, Barbara. *Nickel and Dimed: On (Not) Getting by in America*. New York: Metropolitan Books, 2001.

Eisenberg, Leon, and Leo Kanner, "Early Infantile Autism, 1943–1955." *American Psychiatry Association Research Report* 1 (1957): 556–567.

Ellenby, Whitney. *Autism Uncensored: Pulling Back the Curtain*. Virginia Beach, VA: Köehlerbooks, 2017.

Engber, Daniel. "The Strange Case of Anna Stubblefield." *New York Times Magazine*, October 20, 2015. https://www.New Yorktimes.com/2015/10/25/magazine/the-strange-case-of-anna-stubblefield.html.

Escher, Jill. "Earth to Disability Activists: The Britney Spears Conservatorship Is Irrelevant to Cases of Adults with Severe Autism." *National Council on Severe Autism Blog*, July 28, 2021. https://www.ncsautism.org/blog//earth-to-disability-activists-the-britney-spears-conservatorship-is-irrelevant-to-cases-of-adults-with-severe-autism.

Evans, Bonnie. *The Metamorphosis of Autism: A History of Child Development in Britain* Manchester, UK: Manchester University Press, 2017.

Evans, Elizabeth C. *Physiognomics in the Ancient World*. Philadelphia: American Philosophical Society, 1969.

Eyal, Gil, Brendan Hart, Emine Onculer, et al. *The Autism Matrix: The Social Origins of the Autism Epidemic*. Cambridge, UK: Polity Press, 2010.

Farrow, Ronan, and Jia Tolentino. "Britney Spears's Conservatorship Nightmare." *New Yorker*, July 3, 2021. https://www.newyorker.com/news/american-chronicles/britney-spears-conservatorship-nightmare?gclid=CjwKCAjwgISIBhBfEiwALE19SUbD-fCAwu4VEKMFofpzHmT48Na302Lv9nZnym-BCTNgmB4nGRAVoRoCuNcQAvD_BwE&source=google_sem_dom_promo.

Faure, Patrick, Thierry Legou, and Bruno Gepner. "Evidence of Authorship on Messages in Facilitated Communication: A Case Report Using Accelerometry." *Frontiers in Psychiatry* 11 (December 2020): 543385.

Feinstein, Adam. *A History of Autism: Conversations with the Pioneers*. West Sussex, UK: John Wiley & Sons, 2010.

Ferguson, Philip. "The Social Construction of Mental Retardation." *Social Policy* 18, no. 1 (July 1987): 51–56.

Fevre, Ralph, Amanda Robinson, and Duncan Lewis. "The Ill-Treatment of Employees with Disabilities in British Workplaces." *Work, Employment and Society* 27, no. 2 (2013): 288–307.

Finger, Stanley, and Shawn E. Christ. "Pearl S. Buck and Phenylketonuria (PKU)." *Journal of the History of the Neurosciences* 13, no. 1 (2004): 44–57.

Fisher, James T. "No Search, No Subject? Autism and the American Conversion Narrative." In *Autism and Representation*, edited by Mark Osteen, 51–64. New York: Routledge, 2008.

Fleischer, Doris Zames, and Frieda Zames. *The Disability Rights Movement: From Charity to Confrontation*. Philadelphia: Temple University Press, 2011.

Florance, Cheri. *Maverick Mind: A Mother's Story of Solving the Mystery of Her Unreachable, Unteachable, Silent Son*. New York: G. P. Putnam's Sons, 2004.

Folstein, Susan, and Michael Rutter. "Infantile Autism: A Genetic Study of 21 Twin Pairs." *Journal of Child Psychology and Psychiatry* 18, no. 4 (1977): 297–321.

Forman, Vicki. *This Lovely Life: A Memoir of Premature Motherhood*. Boston: Mariner Books, 2009.

Frank, John P. *My Son's Story*. New York: Alfred A. Knopf, 1952.

Freeman, Melvyn Colin, Kavitha Kolappy, Jose Miguel Caldas de Almeida, et al. "Reversing Hard Won Victories in the Name of Human Rights: A Critique of the General Comment on Article 12 of the UN Convention on the Rights of Persons with Disabilities." *Lancet Psychiatry* 2 (2015): 845–850.

Freitag, Lisa. *Extreme Caregiving: The Moral Work of Raising Children with Special Needs*. New York: Oxford University Press, 2018.

Frith, Uta. "Review: 'Autistic' Children: New Hope for Cure." *Psychological Medicine* 14 (1984): 461–463.

Fromm-Reichmann, Frieda. "Notes on the Development of Treatment of Schizophrenics by Psychoanalytic Psychotherapy." *Psychiatry* 11, no. 3 (1948): 263–273.

Frost, K. Tilden. "I Don't Need or Want Your Autism Awareness." Geek Mom, April 6, 2018. https://geekmom.com/2018/04/i-dont-need-or-want-your-autism-awareness/.

Gant, Sophia. *"One of Those": The Progress of a Mongoloid Child*. New York: Pageant Press, 1957.

Ganz, Jennifer B., Anonis Katsiyannis, and Kristi L. Morin. "Facilitated Communication: The Resurgence of a Disproven Treatment for Individuals with Autism." *Intervention in School and Clinic* 54, no. 1 (2018): 52–56.

Gardner, Martin. "Facilitated Communication: A Cruel Farce." *Skeptical Inquirer* 25, no. 1 (January–February 2001), 17–19.

Garrison, Maxine. *The Angel Spreads Her Wings: The Inspiration of* Angel Unaware *and the Influence of the Roy Rogers Family in the American Home*. Westwood, NJ: Fleming H. Revell, 1956.

General Accounting Office. *Guardianships: Collaboration Needed to Protect Incapacitated Elderly People*. Publication Number GAO-04-655. Washington, DC: GAO, 2004.

Gillberg, Christopher, and Lorna Wing. "Autism: Not an Extremely Rare Disorder." *Acta Psychiatrica* 99 (1999): 399–406.

Gilligan, Carol. *In a Different Voice: Psychological Theory and Women's Development.* Cambridge, MA: Harvard University Press, 1982.

Gilpeer, Valerie, and Emily Grodin. *I Have Been Buried under Years of Dust*. New York: William Morrow, 2021.

Goddard, Henry Herbert. *The Kallikak Family: A Study in the Heredity of Feeble-Mindedness.* New York: Macmillan, 1912.

Goddard, Peyton, and Dianne Peyton, with Carol Cujec. *I Am Intelligent: From Heartbreak to Healing—A Mother and Daughter's Journey through Autism*. Guilford, CT: skirt!, 2012.

Gooding, Piers. *A New Era for Mental Health Law and Policy: Supported Decision-Making and the UN Convention on the Rights of Persons with Disabilities*. Cambridge: Cambridge University Press, 2017.

Green, Gina. "Facilitated Communication: Mental Miracle or Sleight of Hand?" *Behavior and Social Issues* 4, no. 1–2 (1994): 69–85.

Green, Gina. "The Quality of the Evidence." In *Facilitated Communication: The Clinical and Social Phenomenon*, edited by Howard C. Shane, 157–226. San Diego, CA: Singular Press, 1994.

Greenfeld, Josh. *A Child Called Noah: A Family Journey*. New York: Henry Holt, 1972.

Greenfeld, Josh. *A Place for Noah*. New York: Holt, Rinehart and Winston, 1978.

Greenfeld, Karl Taro. *Boy Alone: A Brother's Memoir*. New York: Harper Perennial, 2009.

Gunther, John. *Death Be Not Proud: A Memoir*. New York: Harper & Row, 1949.

HALO (Helping Autism through Learning and Outreach). "Scientific Research into Soma RPM." 2020. https://www.halo-soma.org/research.

Handley, J. B., and Jamison Handley. *Underestimated: An Autism Miracle*. New York: Skyhorse, 2021.

Happé, Francesca G. E. "Understanding Minds and Metaphors: Insights from the Study of Figurative Language in Autism." *Metaphor and Symbolic Activity* 10, no. 4 (1995): 275–295.

Harlow, Harry F., and William T. McKinney. "Nonhuman Primates and Psychoses." *Journal of Autism and Childhood Schizophrenia* 1, no. 4 (1971): 369–375.

Harrington, Anne. "Mother Love and Mental Illness: An Emotional History." *Osiris* 31 (2016): 94–115.

Hart, Charles. *Without Reason: A Family Copes with Two Generations of Autism*. New York: Harper & Row, 1989.

Haskew, Paul, and Anne Donnellan. *Emotional Maturity and Well-Being: Psychological Lessons of Facilitated Communication*. Madison, WI: DRI Press, 1993.

Heard, J. Norman. *Hope through Doing*. New York: John Day, 1968.

Helt, Molly, Elizabeth Kelley, Marcel Kinsbourne, et al. "Can Children with Autism Recover? If So, How?" *Neuropsychology Review* 18 (2008): 339–366.

Hemsley, Bronwyn, Lucy Bryant, Ralf W. Schlosser, et al. "Systematic Review of Facilitated Communication 2014–2018 Finds No New Evidence That Messages Delivered Using Facilitated Communication Are Authored by the Person with Disability." *Autism & Developmental Language Impairments* 3 (2018): 1–8.

Herman, Ellen. "The Siege: The First Eight Years of an Autistic Child, 1967." The Autism History Project. 2019, https://blogs.uoregon.edu/autismhistoryproject/topics/the-siege-1967/.

Hermelin, Beate. *Bright Splinters of the Mind: A Personal Story of Research with Autistic Savants*. London: Jessica Kingsley, 2001.

Higashida, Naoki. *The Reason I Jump*. New York: Random House, 2013.

Hinds, Marcia. *I Know You're in There: Winning Our War against Autism*. New York: Skyhorse, 2020.

Hobson, Matthew, and Nancy Hobson. *I'm So Glad You Found Me in Here*. New York: Ithaca Press, 2010.

Hobson, R. Peter, and Anthony Lee. "Emotion-Related and Abstract Concepts in Autistic People: Evidence from the British Picture Vocabulary Scale." *Journal of Autism and Developmental Disorders* 19 (1989): 601–623.

Hughes, Robert. *Running with Walker*. London: Jessica Kingsley, 2003.

Hughes, Robert. *Walker Finds a Way: Running into the Adult World with Autism*. London: Jessica Kingsley, 2016.

Hundley, Joan Martin. *The Small Outsider: The Story of an Autistic Child*. New York: St. Martin's Press, 1971.

Hutt, C., S. J. Hutt, D. Lee, and C. Ounsted. "Arousal and Childhood Autism." *Nature, London* 204 (1964): 908–909.

I-ASC. "Studying Receptive Language in Nonspeakers through Brain Imaging." 2020. https://i-asc.org/wp-content/uploads/2020/06/2-STUDYING-RECEPTIVE-LANGUAGE-IN-NONSPEAKERS-THROUGH-BRAIN-IMAGING.pdf.

Ingalls, Theodore H. "Etiology of Mongolism: Epidemiologic and Teratologic Implications." *American Journal of Diseases of Children* 74, no. 2 (1947): 147–165.

Ireland, William W. *The Mental Affections of Children: Idiocy, Imbecility and Insanity*. London: J. & A. Churchill, 1898.

Isaacson, Rupert. *The Horse Boy: A Memoir of Healing*. New York: Back Bay Books, 2009.

Iversen, Portia. *Strange Son: Two Mothers, Two Sons, and the Quest to Unlock the Hidden World of Autism*. New York: Riverhead Books, 2006.

Jack, Jordynn. *Autism and Gender: From Refrigerator Mothers to Computer Geeks*. Urbana: University of Chicago Press, 2014.

Jacobson, John W., James A. Mulick, and Allen A. Schwartz. "A History of Facilitated Communication: Science, Pseudoscience, and Antiscience Working Group on Facilitated Communication." *American Psychologist* 50, no. 9 (1995): 750–765.

Jaher, David. *The Witch of Lime Street: Séance, Seduction, and Houdini in the Spirit World*. New York: Broadway Books, 2015.

Jarrett, Simon. *Those They Called Idiots: The Idea of the Disabled Mind from 1700 to the Present Day*. London: Reaktion Books, 2020.

Jaswal, Vikram K., Allison Wayne, and Hudson Golino. "Eye-Tracking Reveals Agency in Assisted Autistic Communication." *Scientific Reports* 10 (2020): 7882. https://www.nature.com/articles/s41598-020-64553-9.

Jewett, Christina. "Nowhere to Go: Young People with Autism Languish in Hospitals." *Kaiser Health News*, September 26, 2017. https://khn.org/news/for-thousands-of-autistic-teens-hospital-ers-serve-as-home/.

Johnson, Carol, and Julia Crowder. *Autism: From Tragedy to Triumph*. Boston: Branden, 1994.

Jones, Kathleen W. "'Mother Made Me Do It': Mother-Blaming and the Women of Child Guidance." In *"Bad" Mothers: The Politics of Blame in Twentieth-Century America*, edited by Molly Ladd-Taylor and Lauri Umansky, 99–126. New York: New York University Press, 1998.

Jones, Kathleen W. *Taming the Troublesome Child: American Families, Child Guidance, and the Limits of Psychiatric Authority*. Cambridge, MA: Harvard University Press, 1999.

Kanner, Leo. "Autistic Disturbances of Affective Contact." *Nervous Child: Journal of Psychopathology, Psychotherapy, Mental Hygiene, and Guidance of the Child* 2 (1943): 217–250.

Kanner, Leo. "Early Infantile Autism Revisited." *Psychiatry Digest* 29, no. 2 (February 1968): 17–28.

Kanner, Leo. *A History of the Care and Study of the Mentally Retarded*. Springfield, IL: Charles C. Thomas, 1964.

Kanner, Leo. *In Defense of Mothers: How to Bring Up Children in Spite of the More Zealous Psychologists*. Springfield, IL: Charles C. Thomas, 1941.

Kanner, Leo. "Problems of Nosology and Psychodynamics of Early Infantile Autism." *Journal of Orthopsychiatry* 19, no. 3 (1949): 416–426.

Kanner, Leo. "To What Extent Is Early Infantile Autism Determined by Constitutional Inadequacies?" *Association for Research in Nervous and Mental Disease* 33, no. 1 (1954): 378–385.

Kaplan, Sarah. "The Millionaire Mom Who Poisoned Her Autistic Son and Called It a Mercy Killing." *Washington Post*, May 29, 2015, https://www.washingtonpost.com/news/morning-mix/wp/2015/05/29/a-murder-or-a-mercy-killing-the-tangled-and-troubling-trial-of-gigi-jordan/.

Kaufman, Barry Neil. *Son-Rise*. New York: Harper & Row, 1976.

Kedar, Ido. *Ido in Autismland: Climbing Out of Autism's Silent Prison*. Self-published, 2012.

Keith, Heather E., and Kenneth D. Keith. *Intellectual Disability: Ethics, Dehumanization, and a New Moral Community*. Malden, MA: Wiley Blackwell, 2013.

Kennedy, Jae, Simi Litvak, and Hale Zukas. "Independent Living and Personal Assistance Services: The Research, Training and Technical Assistance Programs at the World Institute on Disability." *Office of Special Education and Rehabilitation Services* 3 (1994): 43–49.

Kevles, Daniel. *In the Name of Eugenics: Genetics and the Uses of Human Heredity*. Cambridge, MA: Harvard University Press, 1985.

Killilea, Marie. *Karen: A True Story Told by Her Mother*. New York: Open Road Integrated Media, 2018.

Kim, So Hyun, Rhea Paul, Helen Tager-Flusberg, and Catherine Lord. "Language and Communication in Autism." In *Handbook of Autism and Pervasive Developmental Disorders, Vol. 1: Diagnosis, Development, and Brain Mechanisms*, 4th edition, edited by Fred R. Volkmar, Sally J. Rogers, Reha Paul, and Kevin A. Pelphrey. 230–262. Hoboken, NJ: John Wiley & Sons, 2014.

Kirk, Samuel A., Merle B. Karnes, and Winifred D. Kirk. *You and Your Retarded Child: A Manual for Parents of Retarded Children*. New York: Macmillan, 1955.

Kittay, Eva Feder. *Learning from My Daughter: The Value and Care of Disabled Minds*. Oxford: Oxford University Press, 2019.

Kittay, Eva Feder. *Love's Labor: Essays on Women, Equality, and Dependency*. New York: Routledge, 1999.

Kleinman, Arthur. *The Soul of Care: The Moral Education of a Husband and a Doctor*. New York: Viking, 2019.

Kliewer, Christopher, Douglas Biklen, and Amy J. Petersen. "At the End of Intellectual Disability." *Harvard Educational Review* 85, no. 1 (Spring 2015): 1–28.

Knight, Victoria F., Heartley B. Huber, Emily M. Kuntz, et al. "Instructional Practices, Priorities, and Preparedness for Educating Students with Autism and Intellectual Disability." *Focus on Autism and Other Developmental Disabilities* 34, no. 1 (March 2019): 3–14.

Kohn, N. A., J. A. Blumenthal, and A. T. Campbell. "Supported Decision-Making: A Viable Alternative to Guardianship?" *Penn State Law Review* 117 (2013): 1111–1157.

Laughlin, Jason. "Nowhere to Go." *Philadelphia Inquirer*, November 5, 2021. https://www.inquirer.com/health/a/autism-treatment-therapy-care-hospital-health-system-20211105.html.

Law Society of Scotland. "Draft General Comment on Article 12 of the Convention—Equal Recognition Before the Law." November 2013. https://www.ohchr.org/_layouts/15/WopiFrame.aspx?sourcedoc=/Documents/HRBodies/CRPD/GC/LawSocietyOfScotlandArt12.doc&action=default&DefaultItemOpen=1.

League of the Physically Handicapped. *Thesis on Conditions of Physically Handicapped*. J. Paul Leonard Library Digital Collections, UARC_0145, August 1936. http://digital-collections.library.sfsu.edu/digital/collection/p16737coll2/id/994/.

Lee, Carvel. *Tender Tyrant: The Story of a Mentally Retarded Child*. Minneapolis, MN: Augsburg, 1961.

Leone, Marianne. *Jesse: A Mother's Story*. New York: Simon & Schuster, 2010.

Leonnig, Carol D., Lena H. Sun, and Sarah Cohen. "Under Court, Vulnerable Became Victims." *Washington Post*, June 15, 2003. https://www.washingtonpost.com/archive/politics/2003/06/15/under-court-vulnerable-became-victims/859903d5-abc1-4751-8ae6-ab230b8a258e/.

Le-Pape, Jennifer Binder. "An Open Letter to My Son's Skeptics." I-ASC Blog, March 3, 2021. https://i-asc.org/an-open-letter-to-my-sons-skeptics/.

Lerner, Barron H. *When Illness Goes Public: Celebrity Patients and How We Look at Medicine*. Baltimore, MD: Johns Hopkins University Press, 2006.

Levin, Susan. *Unlocked: A Family Emerging from the Shadows of Autism*. New York: Skyhorse, 2015.

Levinson, Abraham. *The Mentally Retarded Child: A Guide for Parents*. New York: John Day, 1952.

Lewiecki-Wilson, Cynthia. "Rethinking Rhetoric through Mental Disabilities." *Rhetoric Review* 22, no. 2 (2003): 156–167.

Lilienfeld, Scott O., Julia Marshall, and James T. Todd. "The Persistence of Fad Interventions in the Face of Negative Scientific Evidence: Facilitated Communication for Autism as a Case Example." *Evidence-Based Communication Assessment and Intervention* 8, no. 2 (2015): 62–101.

Lim, Cynthia. *Wherever You Are: A Memoir of Love, Marriage, and Brain Injury*. Kenmore, WA: Coffeetown Press, 2018.

Linton, Simi. *Claiming Disability: Knowledge and Identity*. New York: New York University Press, 1998.

Liu, Ka-Yuet, Marissa King, and Peter S. Bearman. "Social Influence and the Autism Epidemic." *American Journal of Sociology* 115, no. 5 (March 2010): 1387–1434.

Lombardo, Paul A. *Three Generations, No Imbeciles: Eugenics, the Supreme Court, and* Buck v. Bell. Baltimore, MD: Johns Hopkins University Press, 2008.

London, Matt. "Geraldo: The Story 'Branded on My Soul' That Caused a Revolution." *Fox News*, January 21, 2020. foxnews.com/media/Geraldo-willowbrook-branded-my-soul-fox-nation.

Longmore, Paul K. *Why I Burned My Book: And Other Essays on Disability*. Philadelphia: Temple University Press, 2003.

Longmore, Paul K., and David Goldberger. "The League of the Physically Handicapped and the Great Depression: A Case Study in the New Disability History." *The Journal of American History* 87, no. 3 (December 2000): 888–922.

Lord, Catherine, Eva Petkova, Vanessa Hus, et al. "A Multisite Study of the Clinical Diagnosis of Different Autism Spectrum Disorders." *Archives of General Psychiatry* 69, no. 3 (March 2012): 306–313.

Lovaas, O. Ivar. "Behavioral Treatment and Normal Educational and Intellectual Functioning in Young Autistic Children." *Journal of Consulting and Clinical Psychology* 55, no. 1 (1987): 3–9.

Lutz, Amy S. F. "Baseline." In *We Walk: Life with Severe Autism*, edited by Lutz, 139–152. Ithaca, NY: Cornell University Press, 2020.

Lutz, Amy S. F. *Each Day I Like It Better: Autism, ECT, and the Treatment of Our Most Impaired Children*. Nashville, TN: Vanderbilt University Press, 2014.

Lutz, Amy S. F. "Ideology, Not Data." *Psychology Today* (January 22, 2017). https://www.psychologytoday.com/us/blog/inspectrum/201701/ideology-not-data.

Lutz, Amy S. F. "The Reverse Field of Dreams Fallacy in Disability Policy." *Psychology Today* (November 8, 2021). https://www.psychologytoday.com/us/blog/inspectrum/202111/the-reverse-field-dreams-fallacy-in-disability-policy.

Mahler, Margaret S., Fred Pine, and Anni Bergman. *The Psychological Birth of the Human Infant*. New York: Basic Books, 1975.

Mandell, David S. "A House is Not a Home: The Great Residential Divide in Autism Care." *Autism* 21, no. 7 (September 10, 2017): 810–811. https://journals.sagepub.com/doi/full/10.1177/1362361317722101.

Margolin, Kenneth N. "How Shall Facilitated Communication Be Judged? Facilitated Communication and the Legal System." In *Facilitated Communication: The Clinical and Social Phenomenon,* edited by Howard C. Shane, 227–258. San Diego, CA: Singular Press, 1994.

Martin, Russell. *Out of Silence: A Journey into Language*. New York: Henry Holt, 1994.

Maslin, Abby. *Love You Hard: A Memoir of Marriage, Brain Injury, and Reinventing Love.* New York: Dutton, 2019.

Maurice, Catherine. *Let Me Hear Your Voice: A Family's Triumph over Autism*. New York: Alfred A. Knopf, 1993.

Mazurek, Micah O., Stephen M. Kanne, and Ericka L. Wodka. "Physical Aggression in Children and Adolescents with Autism Spectrum Disorders." *Research in Autism Spectrum Disorders* 7, no. 3 (March 2013): 455–465.

McCarthy, Jenny. *Louder than Words: A Mother's Journey in Healing Autism.* New York: Dutton, 2007.

McDonagh, Patrick, C. F. Goodey, and Tim Stainton. *Intellectual Disability: A Conceptual History, 1200–1900*. Manchester, UK: Manchester University Press, 2018.

McDonnell, Jane Taylor. *News from the Border: A Mother's Memoir of Her Autistic Son.* New York: Ticknor & Fields, 1993.

Melendez, Lyanne. "2 UC Berkeley Students Make History as 1st Nonspeaking Autistic Graduates." *ABC 7 News*, May 19, 2022. https://abc7news.com/uc-berkeley-cal-graduation-nonspeaking-autism-graduates-david-teplitz/11870714/.

Mercier, Charles. *Sanity and Insanity*. London: Walter Scott, 1890.

Milken Institute School of Public Health, Department of Health Policy & Management, George Washington University. "Transitions: A Case Study of the Conversion from Sheltered Workshops to Integrated Employment in Maine." 2015. https://docplayer.net/33593240-Transitions-a-case-study-of-the-conversion-from-sheltered-workshops-to-integrated-employment-in-maine.html.

Minshew, Nancy J., Gerald Goldstein, and Don J. Siegel. "Speech and Language in High-Functioning Autistic Individuals." *Neuropsychology* 9, no. 2 (1995): 255–261.

Mitchell, David T., with Sharon L. Snyder. *The Biopolitics of Disability: Neoliberalism, Ablenationalism, and Peripheral Embodiment*. Ann Arbor: University of Michigan Press, 2015.

Mitchell, David T., and Sharon L. Snyder. *Narrative Prosthesis: Disability and the Dependencies of Discourse*. Ann Arbor: University of Michigan Press, 2000.

Monthie, Jennifer J. "The Myth of Liberty and Justice for All: Guardianship in New York State." *Albany Law Review* 80, no. 3 (2017): 1–41.

Moore, Charlotte. *George and Sam: Two Boys, One Family, and Autism*. New York: St. Martin's Griffin, 2004.

Murphy, Michelle. *The Economization of Life*. Durham, NC: Duke University Press, 2017.

Murray, Dorothy Garst. *This Is Stevie's Story: A Mother's Story of Her Mentally Retarded Son.* Nashville, TN: Abingdon Press, 1956.

Murray, Stuart. *Autism*. New York: Routledge, 2012.

Murray, Stuart. *Representing Autism: Culture, Narrative, Fascination*. Liverpool, UK: Liverpool University Press, 2008.

Nadesan, Majia Holmer. *Constructing Autism: Unravelling the "Truth" and Understanding the Social*. London: Routledge, 2005.

The National Alliance for Caregiving and AARP. "Caregiving in the U.S. 2020." 2020. https://www.caregiving.org/caregiving-in-the-us-2020/.

National Council on Disability. *Beyond Guardianship: Toward Alternatives that Promote Greater Self-Determination*. March 22, 2018. https://ncd.gov/publications/2018/beyond-guardianship-toward-alternatives.

National Disability Rights Network. "Segregated and Exploited: The Failure of the Disability Service System to Provide Quality Work." January 2011. https://www.ndrn.org/wp-content/uploads/2019/03/Segregated-and-Exploited.pdf.

National Institute for Health and Care Excellence. "Autism Spectrum Disorder in Under 19s: Support and Management." June 14, 2021. https://pubmed.ncbi.nlm.nih.gov/34283415/.

Neill, John. "Whatever Became of the Schizophrenogenic Mother?" *American Journal of Psychotherapy* XLIV, no. 4 (October 1990): 499–505.

Ne'eman, Ari. "(Almost) Everything You Need to Know about Sheltered Workshops: Part 2 of 2." *Sometimes a Lion*, September 26, 2015. https://arineeman.com/2015/09/26/sheltered-workshops-part-2/.

Ne'eman, Ari. "Watch the Appointments." *Sometimes a Lion*, January 21, 2017. https://arineeman.com/2017/01/22/watch-the-appointments/.

Nelson, Nathan. *Workshops for the Handicapped in the United States: An Historical and Developmental Perspective*. Springfield, IL: Charles C. Thomas, 1971.

Nichols, Tom. *The Death of Expertise: The Campaign against Established Knowledge and Why It Matters*. Oxford: Oxford University Press, 2017.

Nielsen, Kim E. "Property, Disability, and the Making of the Incompetent Citizen in the United States, 1860s–1940s." In *Disability Histories*, edited by Susan Burch and Michael Rembis, 308–320. Urbana: University of Illinois Press, 2014.

Noll, Steven. *Feeble-Minded in Our Midst: Institutions for the Mentally Retarded in the South, 1900–1940*. Chapel Hill: University of North Carolina Press, 1995.

Nović, Sara. "The Hearing World Must Stop Forcing Deaf Culture to Assimilate." *NBC News*, October 20, 2017. https://www.nbcnews.com/think/opinion/hearing-world-must-stop-forcing-deaf-culture-assimilate-ncna812461.

Olmstead v. L.C. 1999. https://supreme.justia.com/cases/federal/us/527/581/.

O'Neill, Katie, and Rebecca McCarthy. "The Pitfalls of Presumptions." *The ASHA Leader*, December 1, 2018. https://leader.pubs.asha.org/doi/10.1044/leader.FMP.23122018.10.

Orinstein, Alyssa J., Molly Helt, Eva Troyb, et al. "Intervention History of Children and Adolescents with High-Functioning Autism and Optimal Outcomes." *Journal of Developmental & Behavioral Pediatrics* 35, no. 4 (May 2014): 247–256.

Osteen, Mark. *Autism and Representation*. New York: Routledge, 2008.

Ostrolenk, Alexa, Baudouin Forgeot d'Arc, Patricia Jelenic, et al. "Hyperlexia: Systematic Review, Neurocognitive Modelling, and Outcome." *Neuroscience and Biobehavioral Reviews* 79 (2017): 134–149.

Owen-Smith, Ashli A., Stephen Bent, Frances L. Lynch, et al. "Prevalence and Predictors of Complementary and Alternative Medicine Use in a Large Insured Sample of Children with Autism Spectrum Disorders." *Research in Autism Spectrum Disorders* 17 (September 2015): 40–51.

Page, Jordan. "What the Free Britney Movement Did Next." *Vice*, January 20, 2022. https://www.vice.com/en/article/akv78a/when-did-the-free-britney-movement-end.

Palfreman, Jon. "The Australian Origins of Facilitated Communication." In *Facilitated Communication: The Clinical and Social Phenomenon*, edited by Howard C. Shane, 33–56. San Diego, CA: Singular Press, 1994.

Park, Clara Claiborne. *Exiting Nirvana: A Daughter's Life with Autism*. Boston, MA: Back Bay Books, 2001.

Park, Clara Claiborne. *The Siege: A Family's Journey into the World of an Autistic Child*. Boston: Back Bay Books, reissue edition, 1982.

Perske, Robert. "The Dignity of Risk and the Mentally Retarded." *Mental Retardation* 10, no. 1 (1972): 24–27.
Petrocelli, John. *The Life-Changing Science of Detecting Bullshit*. New York: St. Martin's Press, 2021.
Pollak, Richard. *The Creation of Dr. B: A Biography of Bruno Bettelheim*. New York: Simon & Schuster, 1997.
The President's Panel on Mental Retardation. "Report of the Task Force on Law." January 1963. https://mn.gov/mnddc/parallels2/pdf/60s/63/63-ROT-PPMR.pdf.
Price, Margaret. "Defining Mental Disability." In *The Disability Studies Reader*, 4th edition, edited by Lennard J. Davis, 298–307. New York: Routledge, 2013.
Prizant, Barry M., Amy M. Wetherby, Patrick J. Rydell. "Implications of Facilitated Communication for Education and Communication Enhancement Practices for Persons with Autism." In *Facilitated Communication: The Clinical and Social Phenomenon*, edited by Howard C. Shane, 123–156. San Diego, CA: Singular Press, 1994.
Prutsman, Stephen, Autism Society San Francisco Bay Area President. "SFASA Opposition to AB1663." March 7, 2022.
Puar, Jasbir. *The Right to Maim: Debility, Capacity, Disability*. Durham, NC: Duke University Press, 2017.
Quinn, Gerard, and Abigail Rekas-Rosalbo. "Civil Death: Rethinking the Foundations of Legal Personhood for Persons with a Disability." *Irish Jurist* 56 (2016): 286–325.
Rafter, Nicole. "The Criminalization of Mental Retardation." In *Mental Retardation in America: A Historical Reader*, edited by Steven Noll and James W. Trent, Jr., 232–257. New York: New York University Press, 2004.
Radiotimesteam. "Interview: Temple Grandin on Living with Autism." *RadioTimes.com*, April 2, 2011. https://www.radiotimes.com/movies/interview-temple-grandin-on-living-with-autism/.
Rak, Julie. *Boom! Manufacturing Memoir for the Popular Market*. Waterloo, ON: Wilfrid Laurier University Press, 2013.
Rank, Beata. "Adaptation of the Psychoanalytic Technique for the Treatment of Young Children with Atypical Development." *American Journal of Orthopsychiatry* 19, no. 1 (1949): 130–139.
Ribble, Margarethe A. "Disorganizing Factors of Infant Personality." *American Journal of Psychiatry* 98, no. 3 (1941): 459–463.
Rimland, Bernard. *Infantile Autism*. New York: Appleton-Century-Crofts, 1964.
Roberts, Nancy. *David*. Richmond, VA: John Knox Press, 1968.
Robison, John Elder. "Does Mom Know Best, or Do We Presume Autistic Competence?" *Psychology Today* (January 22, 2016). https://www.psychologytoday.com/us/blog/my-life-aspergers/201601/does-mom-know-best-or-do-we-presume-autistic-competence.
Rogers, Dale Evans. *Angel Unaware: A Touching Story of Love and Loss, 50th Anniversary Edition*. Grand Rapids, MI: Revell, 2004.
"Rogers Guardianship." Mass.gov. https://www.mass.gov/rogers-guardianships.
Rose, Sarah F. *No Right to Be Idle: The Invention of Disability, 1840s–1930s*. Chapel Hill: University of North Carolina Press, 2017.
Rothenberg, Mira, and Homer Page. "The Rebirth of Jonny." *Harper's Magazine* 220, no. 1317 (February 1, 1960): 57–66.
Rundblad, Gabriella, and Dagmara Annaz. "The Atypical Development of Metaphor and Metonymy Comprehension in Children with Autism." *Autism: The International Journal of Research and Practice* 14, no. 1 (2010): 29–46.
Rutter, Michael. "Autistic Children: Infancy to Adulthood." *Seminars in Psychiatry* 2 (1970): 435–450.
Rutter, Michael. "Concepts of Autism: A Review of Research." *Journal of Child Psychology and Psychiatry* 9 (1968): 1–25.

Rutter, Michael. "Medical Aspects of the Education of Psychotic (Autistic) Children." In *Some Approaches to Teaching Autistic Children: A Collection of Papers*, edited by P. T. B. Weston, 61–74. Oxford: Pergamon Press, 1965.

Rutter, M., D. Greenfeld, and L. Lockyer. "A Five to Fifteen-Year Follow-Up Study of Infantile Psychosis." *British Journal of Psychiatry* 113 (1967): 1183–1199.

Sarris, Marina. "Antipsychotics and Autism: Weighing the Benefits, Eyeing the Risks." *Interactive Autism Network*, December 13, 2016. https://iancommunity.org/ssc/antipsychotics-and-autism-weighing-benefits-eyeing-risks.

SARTAC. "The Process of Terminating Guardianship Using Supported Decision Making." April 27, 2020. https://www.youtube.com/watch?v=PmWAZpItZ6Q.

Savarese, Ralph. *Reasonable People: A Memoir of Autism and Adoption*. New York: Other Press, 2007.

Schaefer, Nicola. *Does She Know She's There?* Markham, ON: Fitzhenry and Whiteside, 1999.

Schain, Richard J., and Daniel X. Freedman. "Studies on 5-Hydroxyindole Metabolism in Autistic and Other Mentally Retarded Children." *Journal of Pediatrics* 58 (March 1961): 315–320.

Scheibel, Gretchen, Thomas L. Zane, and Kathleen N. Zimmerman. "An Economic Evaluation of Emerging and Ineffective Interventions: Examining the Role of Cost When Translating Research into Practice." *Exceptional Children* 88, no. 3 (January 20, 2022): 245–262.

Schlosser, Ralf W., Susan Balandin, Bronwyn Hemsley, et al. "Facilitated Communication and Authorship: A Systematic Review." *Augmentative and Alternative Communication* 30, no. 4 (2014): 359–368.

Schmalzreid, B. R., Sr. *Sunshine: A Slow Miracle*. Boston, MA: Daughter of St. Paul, 1965.

Schopler, Eric. "Parents of Autistic Children as Scapegoats." *Journal of Contemporary Psychotherapy* 4, no. 1 (Winter 1971): 17–22.

Schreibman, Laura. *The Science and Fiction of Autism*. Cambridge, MA: Harvard University Press, 2005.

Schroeder, Elizabeth. "The Right to Decide: Developments in North American Guardianship Law." *GW Law International Law and Policy Brief* (March 21, 2022). https://studentbriefs.law.gwu.edu/ilpb/2022/03/21/the-right-to-decide-developments-in-north-american-guardianship-law-2/.

Scotch, Richard K. *From Good Will to Civil Rights: Transforming Federal Disability Policy*. Philadelphia: Temple University Press, 1984.

Seroussi, Karyn. *Unraveling the Mystery of Autism and Pervasive Developmental Disorder: A Mother's Story of Research and Recovery*. New York: Simon and Schuster, 2000.

Shakespeare, Tom. *Disability Rights and Wrongs Revisited*. New York: Routledge, 2006.

Shakespeare, Tom. "The Social Model of Disability." In *The Disability Studies Reader*, 4th edition, edited by Lennard J. Davis, 214–221. New York: Routledge, 2013.

Shane, Howard C. "Establishing the Source of Communication." In *Facilitated Communication: The Clinical and Social Phenomenon*, edited by Howard C. Shane, 259–298. San Diego, CA: Singular Press, 1994.

Shane, Howard C. "Facilitated Communication: Factual, Fictional, or Factitious." In *Facilitated Communication: The Clinical and Social Phenomenon*, edited by Howard C. Shane, 1–32. San Diego, CA: Singular Press, 1994.

Shane, Howard C. "The Facilitated Nightmare: The Dark Side of the Phenomenon." In *Facilitated Communication: The Clinical and Social Phenomenon*, edited by Howard C. Shane, 299–319. San Diego, CA: Singular Press, 1994.

Shapiro, Joseph P. *No Pity: People with Disabilities Forging a New Civil Rights Movement*. New York: Three Rivers Press, 1993.

Shechner, Mark. "A Superstar Psychologist Unmasked as the Dean of Deception." *The Buffalo News*, January 12, 1997. https://buffalonews.com/news/a-superstar-psychologist-unmasked-as-the-dean-of-deception/article_5bcca57f-699e-5547–93a9–119ac22c0246.html/.

Sheffer, Edith. *Asperger's Children: The Origins of Autism in Nazi Vienna*. New York: W. W. Norton, 2018.

Shogren, Karrie A., Michael L. Wehmeyer, Heather Lassman, and Anjali J. Forber-Pratt. "Supported Decision Making." *Education and Training in Autism and Developmental Disabilities* 52, no. 2 (June 2017): 144–157.

Siegel, Bryna. *The Politics of Autism*. Oxford: Oxford University Press, 2018.

Sienkiewicz-Mercer, Ruth, and Steven B. Kaplan. *I Raise My Eyes to Say Yes*. West Hartford, CT: Whole Health Books, 1989.

Silberman, Steve. *Neurotribes: The Legacy of Autism and the Future of Neurodiversity*. New York: Avery, 2015.

Silverman, Chloe. *Understanding Autism: Parents, Doctors, and the History of a Disorder*. Princeton, NJ: Princeton University Press, 2012.

Simmons, William Paul, Janyce Boynton, and Todd Landman. "Facilitated Communication, Neurodiversity, and Human Rights." *Human Rights Quarterly* 43, no. 1 (February 2021): 138–167.

Simplican, Stacy Clifford. *The Capacity Contract: Intellectual Disability and the Question of Citizenship*. Minneapolis: University of Minnesota Press, 2015.

Sinclair, Jim. "Don't Mourn for Us." *Autonomy, the Critical Journal of Interdisciplinary Autism Studies* 1, no. 1 (October 2012): 1–4.

Singer, Alison, Amy Lutz, Jill Escher, and Alycia Halladay. "A Full Semantic Toolbox Is Essential for Autism Research and Practice to Thrive." *Autism Research* 16 (2023): 497–501. https://onlinelibrary.wiley.com/doi/epdf/10.1002/aur.2876.

Singer, Judy. *Odd People In: The Birth of Community amongst People on the "Autistic Spectrum": A Personal Exploration of a New Social Movement Based on Neurological Diversity*. A thesis presented to the faculty of Humanities and Social Sciences in partial fulfillment of the requirements for the degree of Bachelor of Arts Social Science (Honours), Faculty of Humanities and Social Science, University of Technology, Sydney: 1988.

Singh, Jennifer S. *Multiple Autisms: Spectrums of Advocacy and Genomic Science*. Minneapolis: University of Minnesota Press, 2016.

Smith, J. David, and Michael L. Wehmeyer. "Who Was Deborah Kallikak?" *Intellectual and Developmental Disabilities* 50, no. 2 (2012): 169–178.

Sousa, Amy. "From Refrigerator Mothers to Warrior-Heroes: The Cultural Identity Transformation of Mothers Raising Children with Intellectual Disabilities." *Symbolic Interaction* 34, no. 2 (2011): 220–243.

Spreat, Scott, and James William Conroy. "Longitudinal Investigation of Vocational Engagement." *Journal of Policy and Practice in Intellectual Disabilities* 12, no. 4 (December 2015): 266–271.

Stacey, Patricia. *The Boy Who Loved Windows: Opening the Heart and Mind of a Child Threatened with Autism*. Cambridge, MA: Da Capo Press, 2003.

Stafford, Stephen. "Nothing Less than the Minimum: People with Disabilities Should Not Earn Less than Minimum Wage." *University of Cincinnati Law Review* (December 27, 2021). https://uclawreview.org/2021/12/27/nothing-less-than-the-minimum-people-with-disabilities-should-not-earn-less-than-minimum-wage/.

Starr, Paul. *The Social Transformation of American Medicine*. New York: Basic Books, 1982.

Stehli, Annabel. *The Sound of a Miracle: A Child's Triumph over Autism*. New York: Doubleday, 1991.

Stout, Lucille. *I Reclaimed My Child: The Story of a Family into Which a Retarded Child Was Born*. Philadelphia: Chilton, 1959.

Strecker, Edward A. *Their Mothers' Sons: The Psychiatrist Examines an American Problem*. Philadelphia: J. B. Lippincott, 1946.

Sultan, Reina. "The Horror of an Unwanted Conservatorship According to People Who Lived It." *Vice*, July 8, 2021. https://www.vice.com/en/article/epn57n/what-its-like-to-live-under-a-conservatorship-or-guardianship-britney-spears.

Sundstrom, Kathy. "Carer: 'I Fell in Love': Grandma Guilty of Indecent Dealing." *Sunshine Coast Daily*, October 16, 2014. www.couriermail.com.au%2Fnews%2Fqueensland%2Fsunshine-coast%2Fi-love-him-disability-carer-faces-court-over-love-affair%2Fnews-.

Swadron, Barry. *Mental Retardation—the Law—Guardianship*. ON: National Institute on Mental Retardation, 1972.

Tager-Flusberg, Helen. "Autistic Children's Talk about Psychological States: Deficits in the Early Acquisition of a Theory of Mind." *Child Development* 63 (1992): 161–172.

Taylor, Lori Ashley. *Dragonfly: A Daughter's Emergence from Autism*. New York: Skyhorse, 2018.

Teaster, Pamela B., Erica F. Wood, Naomi Karp, et al. *Wards of the State: A National Study of Public Guardianship*. Chicago, IL: The Retirement Research Foundation, 2005. https://www.americanbar.org/content/dam/aba/administrative/law_aging/wardofstatefinal.pdf.

Tinbergen, Nikolaas. "Ethology and Stress Diseases." *Science* 185, no. 4145 (July 5, 1974): 20–27.

Tinbergen, Nikolaas, and Elisabeth A. Tinbergen. *"Autistic" Children: New Hope for a Cure*. London; Boston; Sydney: George Allen & Unwin, 1983.

Tino, Gregory C. *The Autistic Mind Finally Speaks: Letterboard Thoughts*. Independently published, 2020.

Travers, Jason, and Kevin M. Ayres. "A Critique of Presuming Competence of Learners with Autism or Other Developmental Disabilities." *Education and Training in Autism and Developmental Disabilities* 50, no. 4 (December 2015): 371–387.

Treffert, Darold A. "Dying with Their Rights On." *American Journal of Psychiatry* 130, no. 9 (September 1973): 1041.

Trent, James. *Inventing the Feeble Mind: A History of Mental Retardation in the United States*. Berkeley: University of California Press, 1994.

Tronto, Joan C. *Moral Boundaries: A Political Argument for an Ethic of Care*. New York: Routledge, 1993.

Tucker, Charlotte D. *Betty Lee: Care of Handicapped Children*. New York: Macmillan, 1954.

Tustin, Frances. *Autism and Childhood Psychosis*. London: Hogarth, 1972.

Tustin, Frances. *Autistic States in Children*. London: Routledge, 1992.

Twachtman-Cullen, Diane. *A Passion to Believe: Autism and the Facilitated Communication Phenomenon*. Boulder, CO: Westview Press, 1997.

Tyor, Peter L., and Leland V. Bell. *Caring for the Retarded in America: A History*. Westport, CT: Greenwood Press, 1984.

United for Communication Choice press release. July 2018. https://unitedforcommunicationchoice.org/national-coalition-opposes-ashas-attempts-to-restrict-communication-choice/950/.

United Nations. *Convention on the Rights of Persons with Disabilities*. 2006. https://www.un.org/development/desa/disabilities/convention-on-the-rights-of-persons-with-disabilities.html.

United Nations. Convention on the Rights of Persons with Disabilities (2006), Article 12. https://www.un.org/development/desa/disabilities/convention-on-the-rights-of-persons-with-disabilities/article-12-equal-recognition-before-the-law.html.

United Nations. "Declaration on the Rights of Mentally Retarded Persons." December 20, 1971. https://www.ohchr.org/en/instruments-mechanisms/instruments/declaration-rights-mentally-retarded-persons.

United Nations. World Autism Day 2017. http://webtv.un.org/search/toward-autonomy-and-self-determination-world-autism-awareness-day-2017/5380816054001?term=world%20autism%20awareness%20day%202017.

United States Commission on Civil Rights. "Subminimum Wages: Impacts on the Civil Rights of People with Disabilities." September 2020. https://www.usccr.gov/files/2020/2020-09-17-Subminimum-Wages-Report.pdf.

van der Horst, Frank C. P. *John Bowlby: From Psychoanalysis to Ethology*. West Sussex, UK: Wiley-Blackwell, 2011.

van Rosmalen, Lenny, René van der Veer, and Frank C. P. van der Horst. "The Nature of Love: Harlow, Bowlby and Bettelheim on Affectionless Mothers." *History of Psychiatry* 31, no. 2 (2020): 227–231.

Vicedo, Marga. *Intelligent Love: The Story of Clara Park, Her Autistic Daughter, and the Myth of the Refrigerator Mother*. Boston: Beacon Press, 2021.

Vicedo, Marga. *The Nature and Nurture of Love: Imprinting to Attachment in Cold War America*. Chicago: University of Chicago Press, 2013.

Vogt, Evon Z., and Ray Hyman. *Water Witching U.S.A.* Chicago: University of Chicago Press, 1959.

Vyse, Stuart. "Of Eye Movements and Autism: The Latest Chapter in a Continuing Controversy." *Skeptical Inquirer* (May 30, 2020) https://skepticalinquirer.org/exclusive/of-eye-movements-and-autism-the-latest-chapter-in-a-continuing-controversy/.

Waltz, Mitzi. *Autism: A Social and Medical History*. Hampshire, UK: Palgrave Macmillan, 2013.

Warren, Zachary, Jeremy Veenstra-VanderWeele, Wendy Stone, et al. *Therapies for Children with Autism Spectrum Disorders: Comparative Effectiveness Review No. 26*. Rockville, MD: Agency for Healthcare Research and Quality, 2011.

Washington, Kate. *Already Toast: Caregiving and Burnout in America*. Boston: Beacon Press, 2021.

Wehmeyer, Michael L., and Robert L. Schalock. "The Parent Movement: Late Modern Times (1950 CE to 1980 CE)." In *The Story of Intellectual Disability: An Evolution of Meaning, Understanding, and Public Perception*, edited by Michael L. Wehmeyer, 187–232. Baltimore, MD: Paul H. Brookes, 2013.

Weisman, Aly. "Jenny McCarthy Slams 'Irresponsible' Rumor Her Son Was Misdiagnosed with Autism." *Business Insider*, January 6, 2014. https://www.businessinsider.com/jenny-mccarthy-slams-rumors-her-son-was-misdiagnosed-with-autism-2014-1.

Weiss, Michael, J. Salomon, and Sheldon H. Wagner. "Emerging Validation of Facilitated Communication: New Findings about Old Assumptions." In *Contested Words, Contested Science: Unraveling the Facilitated Communication Controversy*, edited by Douglas Biklen and Donald N. Cardinal, 135–156. New York: Teachers College Press, 1997.

Whelan, Michael. "Inspiration if Power: Voices of Information and Advocacy for the Reader of Autism Narratives." *Social Alternatives* 36, no. 4 (2017): 44–49.

Wing, Lorna. "Asperger's Syndrome: A Clinical Account." *Psychological Medicine* 11 (1981): 115–129.

Wing, Lorna. *Children Apart: Autistic Children and Their Families*. London, UK: British Medical Association in conjunction with the National Association for Mental Health, 1970.

Wing, Lorna. "Reflections on Opening Pandora's Box." *Journal of Autism and Developmental Disorders* 35, no. 2 (April 2005): 197–203.

Wing, Lorna. "Severe Impairments of Social Interaction and Associated Abnormalities in Children: Epidemiology and Classification." *Journal of Autism and Developmental Disorders* 9, no. 1 (1979): 11–29.

Wolfensberger, Wolf. "The 'Facilitated Communication' Craze as an Instance of Pathological Science: The Cold Fusion of Human Services." In *Facilitated Communication: The Clinical and Social Phenomenon*, edited by Howard C. Shane, 57–122. San Diego, CA: Singular Press, 1994.

Wolfensberger, Wolf, Bengt Nirje, and Simon Olshansky. *The Principle of Normalization in Human Services*. Toronto, ON: National Institute on Mental Retardation, 1972.

Wright, David. *Downs: The History of a Disability*. Oxford: Oxford University Press, 2011.

Wylie, Philip. *Generations of Vipers*. New York: Farrar & Rinehart, 1942.

Zelizer, Viviana A. *Pricing the Priceless Child*. New York: Basic Books, Inc., 1985.

Zenderland, Leila. "The Parable of *The Kallikak Family:* Explaining the Meaning of Heredity in 1912." In *Mental Retardation in America: A Historical Reader*, edited by Steven Noll and James W. Trent, Jr., 165–185. New York: New York University Press, 2004.

Zuber, Andrea, and Julia Burkstaller. "Letter to Members of the Senate Human Services Reform Finance and Policy Committee." November 10, 2021. https://www.senate.mn/committees/2021-2022/3096_Committee_on_Human_Services_Reform_Finance_and_Policy/The%20Arc%20Minnesota%20Subminimum%20Wage%20Written%20Testimo New York%2011.10.21.pdf.

Index

For the benefit of digital users, indexed terms that span two pages (e.g., 52–53) may, on occasion, appear on only one of those pages.